Medicine from the Trees

To Coco, Tommy, and Brian,
who continue to ground
me while we all grow
upward, together.

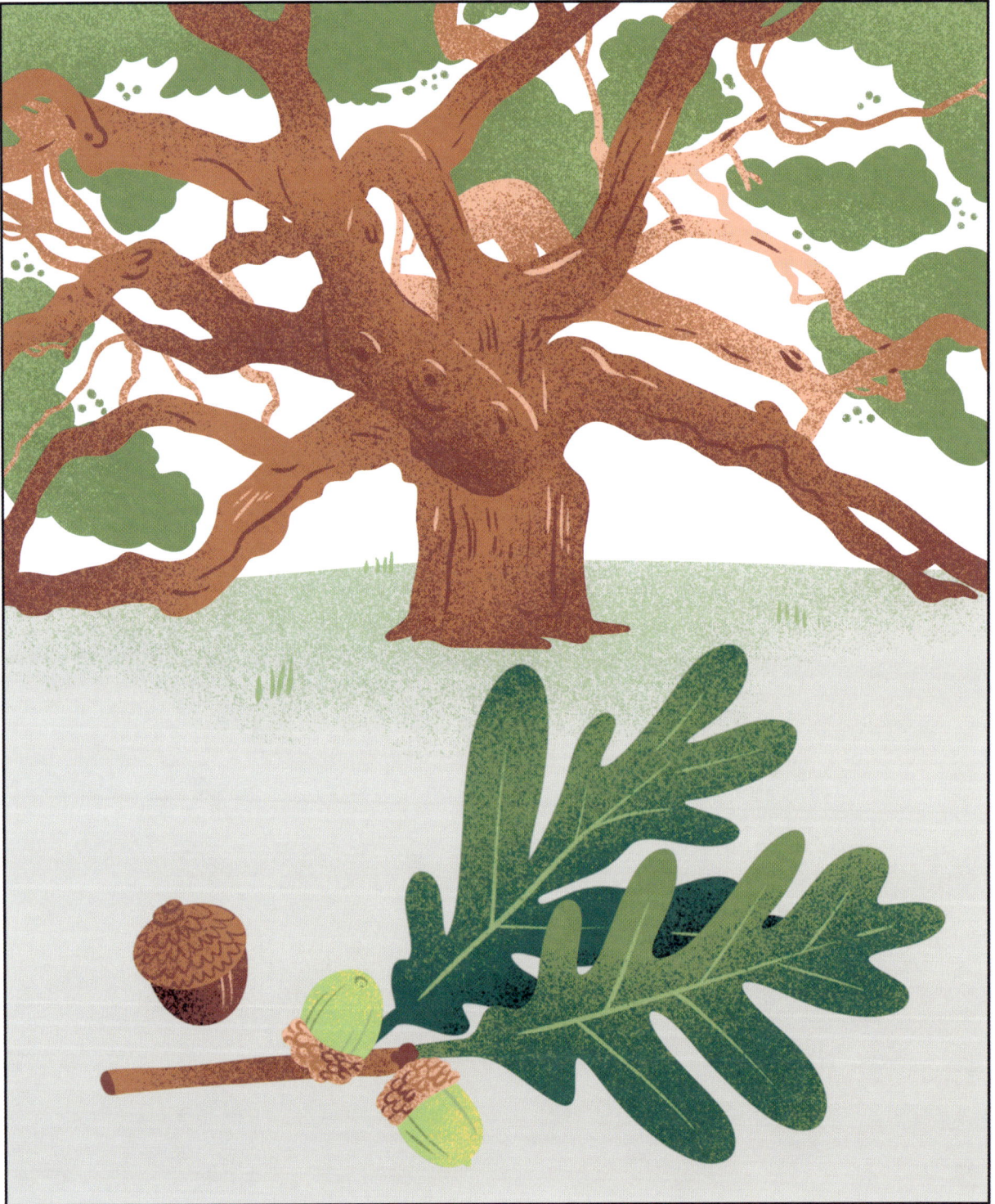

Dr. JJ Pursell

Medicine from the Trees

Herbal Remedies from the
Forest for Whole-Body
Health and Wellness

RIZZOLI
NEW YORK

New York · Paris · London · Milan

First published in the United States of America in 2026 by
Rizzoli International Publications, Inc.
49 West 27th Street
New York, NY 10001
www.rizzoliusa.com

Publisher: Charles Miers
Editor: Stacee Gravelle Lawrence
Design: 508 Creative
Production Manager: Colin Hough Trapp
Managing Editor: Lynn Scrabis

ISBN: 978-0-8478-7611-2
Library of Congress Control Number: 2025941940

Printed in China
2026 2027 2028 / 10 9 8 7 6 5 4 3 2 1

The authorized representative in the EU for product safety and
compliance is Mondadori Libri S.p.A., via Gian Battista Vico 42,
Milan, Italy, 20123, www.mondadori.it.

Visit us online:
Instagram: @RizzoliBooks
Facebook.com/RizzoliNewYork
Youtube.com/user/RizzoliNY

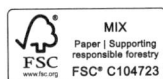

MIX
Paper | Supporting
responsible forestry
FSC
www.fsc.org   FSC® C104723

Contents

Introduction

Through the years, I've noticed a shift in how I enter the woods. As a child, I recognized pure joy as I ran down dirt pathways marked as trails. As a teenager, hikes in the woods often felt like forced activity, but one I would inevitably surrender to as my pounding footsteps fell into a rhythm. When I was muddling through early adulthood, the forest became a place of refuge in which I could breathe and escape whatever drama seemed to be drowning my existence. Now, as I inch toward becoming the definition of an "elder," I'm aware that something in my brain and body shifts as I get closer to the trees. As I turn off a main road and into the woods, my senses become almost preternaturally heightened. Like a dog who knows it's about to experience total unleashed freedom, my body seems to become more alive the moment I park my car. Immediately I take in the canopies of greens that summoned me, the musky scent of the earth. No matter what time of year it is, this scent infuses my brain and triggers the remembrance of a feeling I associate with "home." At this point my scientist brain (without fail) plays its automated message reminding me that a lot of these scents are derived from the monoterpenes emitted by the conifer and broad-leafed trees. These are volatile oils, or more simply put, the oils in the trees that make them smell like they do. Maybe it's as simple as recent clinical studies have shown: monoterpenes have a chemical effect on the brain that make humans feel at peace in the forest. Maybe not.

From the moment I get out of my car, it is as though time stops. I am no longer concerned with the day's previous events, or the to-do list waiting for me. It is only the now, standing here, surrounded by every color the earth can create that matters. I breathe in and out, filling my lungs with a sense of gratitude. Why am I feeling grace? Upon reflection, I believe it is because here, in the forest, I am reminded of my truest self. Not the doctor, or the mom, or any of the other hundred-and-one roles I seem to play in my life. The forest is a place I come to feel alive, to saturate my being if only for a little while with a sense that everything is right in the world.

While you might have personally felt that there are benefits to spending time in nature yourself, it has now been scientifically proven. It measurably boosts clarity in thinking, relaxes muscle tension, improves sleep, reduces heart disease, improves mental health, and lowers cortisol levels. Monoterpenes have been shown to reduce instances of asthma, atopic dermatitis, and to provide the brain with neuroprotective support.

Spending as little as ten minutes a day outside has been shown to have positive effects. A study performed in Denmark examined 900,000 residents born between 1985 and 2003 and found that children who lived in neighborhoods with more green space had a reduced risk of mental disorders later in life. Forest bathing, the act of slowly walking through the woods and actively taking in all of the sounds, sights, smells, and tactility of your surroundings has also been actively studied in recent years. Japan is one of the countries where the forest usage programs for human health have been well developed. The forest agency of the Japanese government introduced the term *shinrin-yoku*, defined as "taking in the forest atmosphere, or forest bathing" in 1982, and instituted a "therapeutic effects of forests plan" in 2005. The results are in, and it's all good. The potential to lower blood pressure, boost immunity, and lift the mood is just waiting to be had from an activity that is so very simple.

Even though I've walked many of my familiar nearby trails a hundred times over, my eyes perpetually scan and inevitably find something new every trip. Perhaps a tree that has silently fallen and been caught by another, the spread of moss creeping along a log that marks the trail's edge, indicating that water has for some reason decided to divert off its normal path. These simple things mark life's cycles and the passage of time for me and in some way, my relationship to both. Woods and forests are inclusive of an incredible amount of life, each entity playing a vital role in the sustainability of the whole environment. But it is the trees that, time after time, draw me in. These stately, magical, gnarly, twisted, and distinctly unique creatures— sapling or old growth—all manage to coexist. They're absolutely integral to our human world. In David Abram's book *The Spell of the Sensuous*, he describes a universal language that was once shared by everyone and everything of this world. One common language that everything shared, from the wind to the trees, animals, humans, and plants. This language provided the ability to exchange knowledge through equality. There was no hierarchy. All was in balance, and all was valued. My thoughts often wander to theories that try to explain why there's been a shift in that relationship, and the evolution of humans' relationships with trees post-shift. Why do some populations have little regard for these living entities, ripping them from the ground to accommodate human designs for other plans, while others have traditions that have revered trees throughout time? Endless questions abound in my mind: What caused some populations to lose a belief that trees were spiritually valuable? If some of the religious texts that have formed the basis for much of Western philosophy state the importance of trees, why did they not remain honored in the Western world? Why do we feel better after walking in the woods? How far and wide does the "wood wide web" go? Is it a coincidence that the human respiratory system is photosynthesis in reverse?

Poets such as Hermann Hesse and Mary Oliver write about forests as revered places, a place where one can feel connected to the spirit, however you define it. Throughout history, cultures have marked sacred trees and formed natural sanctuaries, across the globe. Bodhi, fig, and oak trees are good examples. A bounty of books, poems, and art have been dedicated to the endeavors of attempting to better understand our connection to nature, but in particular, what it is that just makes us feel so good after spending time in it. Daoist principles state that staying rooted within the cosmos of our microcosm will set us free by keeping us grounded. When I reflect on this principle, my mind always conjures a vision of a tree with its roots reaching to the center of the earth. In my mind, I might see my beloved childhood willow, or the multicolored eucalyptus in Peru, but the mental image always reminds me to breathe and stay rooted. Through this meditation of sorts, I've realized the impact that trees have made in my life. Much like a protective grandmother or an overzealous aunt who is always up in your business, various trees have rooted themselves in the timeline of my existence. This

curiosity about the workings of my own mind, as well as my love for botanical medicine, quickly became the spark that led to the creation of this book.

In the following pages you will find thirty-four tree stories, each a personal reflection of how a given species has featured as part of my own life's timeline. Following each story, there is a page which describes how to use each tree medicinally as well as how to grow it. If you've read any of my other books, this part of the format will look somewhat familiar to you. Lastly, each featured tree includes recipes for how you might incorporate that unique tree's uniquely medicinal attributes into your own life. Instead of focusing solely on recipes that can build up your herbal medicine cabinet, I've curated a fun collection of recipes to inspire the mind to incorporate tree medicine into your regular daily routines.

My hope, as always, is to stimulate your interest in botanical medicine and to help you care for yourself and your family. But a prayer is also infused in the pages of this book—a prayer that we all make time to pause and give thanks to the mighty beings around us commonly referred to as trees. To simply acknowledge the trees in your neighborhood, communities, and perhaps backyard. To give thanks for the clean air they provide and the balance they create in our ecosystem. And lastly, should the need arise, that we will all come together and protect them.

—*Dr. JJ Pursell*

Making Tree Medicine

Making medicines from plants is based on ancient wisdom. A knowledge that at one time was passed down from generation to generation and deeply ingrained into the daily practices of many cultures. We can find proof of its existence on Sumerian tablets, Egyptian papyrus, cave art in France, and in the scrolls of China. But even before the first written documentation, there was the witnessing of practical application and the transferring of information through oral history. Families with knowledge of how and when to use certain plants to heal wounds or fight fevers possessed one of the highest types of commodity: survival.

I didn't have a grandmother from the Old World who knew these ways, but once I began to study herbalism it was like a sort of collective memory was switched on inside me. Learning the basics of herbal dynamics, such as the effects of a demulcent or how to identify an astringent by taste, felt like second nature. For the first time I felt connected to *something*, an origin place that provided me peace, comfort, and confidence. I've heard similar stories from students over the years—how herbal medicine information didn't necessarily feel new to them, but as if it was awakening after a long sleep.

As we are now learning, DNA consists of much more than a record of our physical traits. Therefore, I think it is more than reasonable to consider that ancestral knowledge can be passed down through generations at a cellular level. One of my early mentors, Linda Quintana, used to say that when we take in an herb, particularly one that is readily found and foraged across the globe, that our bodies remember its taste and function on a cellular level, too, providing recognition and action for the body. I love thinking about that when I cut and eat some chickweed from my garden. Is it possible that the chickweed on my salad triggers a part of my DNA that remembers my ancestors eating chickweed thousands of years ago?

Making plant medicines, to my mind, can awaken that same familiarity. Even the simple act of cutting a few small stems of yarrow and adding hot water to make a tea can elicit a reconnection point. In recent years there has been a resurgence in the power of plant medicine and earth healing. New books and articles on forest bathing,

ion principles, herbal traditions, and earth grounding all remind us that connecting to the earth and the environment around us is just as important as connecting with other humans. Making herbal medicines is a bridge to both. I connect with the earth as I gather the healing plants and establish connection through the art of making medicine. Two tasks that are as old as the beginning of time.

Here is what I suggest in order to awaken your relationship with botanical medicine. First, find an herb that grows right around your house. Naturally you'll want to ensure it is free and clear of fertilizers or herbicides. Then, find a comfortable spot next to the plant and try to meditate for five or ten minutes. Getting present in that space will do wonders for opening up your intuition and inner listening skills. By sitting still, you might be lucky enough to have the herb tell you a story or offer up its medicinal knowledge. This experience alone has taught me more than most herb books.

Next, you'll want to look at the plant and do your best to correctly identify it. You can use books, the internet, or a tool like Google Lens. Correct identification is key but so is a healthy specimen. Does it look vibrant and full of life? If so, you are on the right track. Next, consider what color it is and what it looks like. As part of the process, it is best to write down all your thoughts in an herb journal and perhaps sketch a little picture of it. Then, take a little pinch of it and smell it. Does it smell sweet? Sharp? What does it remind you of? Does it evoke any memories? Write all of this down, even if it seems unformed or superfluous. The next part of the process is to make a cup of tea. Put a little sprig in a cup and pour hot water over it. Let it steep for a few minutes. While it is steeping, be sure to hold the cup under your nose and inhale the steam. What does this smell like? We often describe tea smells as grassy, strong, minty, or earthy. After you've written down your thoughts on smell, take a drink. What does it taste like? Does it have a flavor or quality? When you drink it, how does it make your body feel? Where does it seem to travel to in your body? Even though it is a warm cup of tea, does it make you feel hot, or does it cool you down? Going through this process gives you an immense amount of information and forms the building blocks of an herbal relationship. It is also one of the best ways to strengthen inner confidence and intuition as a budding herbalist.

TYPES OF MEDICINE YOU CAN MAKE FROM TREES

In the recipe section for each tree in this volume, I've offered up unique recipes with clear instructions. This section on the other hand, is to remind you that, depending on the part of the tree we use, you can make any of the following medicine types as well.

The most common, and easiest, form of herbal medicine is tea. Collect a few needles, flowers, or a bit of bark and you can have medicinal tea in minutes. Herbal syrups can be produced with little to no cooking skills, and making an herbal oil is also a very simple process. Salves for topical use can be made quickly and poultices, fomentations, and herbal capsules are all easily attainable even for the inexperienced. Below I will go through each one to help familiarize yourself with the terminology and techniques.

TEA

When we make herbal tea, the first thing we need to consider is what part of the tree we are using. Typically the parts of the tree we might use are the needles, leaves, buds, flowers, seeds, and bark. The needles, leaves, buds and flowers are of a more delicate matter, which means they should be infused when making tea. This is in comparison to the seeds and bark, which often need to be decocted, or boiled, to release the medicinal qualities into the water.

An infusion, the soaking of herbal material in hot water, can be made by the cup, or in larger quantities and consumed over two or three days. When you are using herbs to actively rebalance function in the body, drinking two to three cups per day for several weeks is often required. Herbal medicine is a slow and steady reorganization of dysfunction. It takes time to unpack the twists and turns of a knotted imbalance and return it to its healthy track. Keep in mind, if you have a chronic dysfunction, you likely realize it didn't just come on suddenly. It often took months or even years of slow building to physically reach the havoc it causes your body today. To reestablish health means you need to backtrack. What I mean is this: if it was a two-year process of dysfunction, it can easily take just as long to get back to baseline. With herbal medicines you typically feel relief of symptoms quite quickly, unweaving all of the damage that the dysfunction created takes time. *Infusion by the cup:* Place herbs in a cup or tea strainer and pour (almost) boiling water over. Let it infuse for 8 to 10 minutes, unless you are working with a plant with a high bitter principle, such as hops, then just 3 to 4 minutes.

Decoction: Decoction is the simmering of heavy herbal materials such as roots, seeds, and barks. Place 2 cups of water in a saucepan and 1 tablespoon of herbs. Bring to a simmer and simmer for 10 to 15 minutes with lid ajar. Strain into a tea mug.

Medicinal-strength brew: I often make a 32-oz. mason jar of herbal tea when I know I want to drink 2 or 3 cups per day. This is basically an infusion process, but let the herbs infuse for over 4 hours. This is particularly handy if you have a blend that has both bark and needles, for example. Due to the long infusion time, the medicinal elements will be drawn from the plant material that normally would need to be simmered.

Put 4 or 5 tablespoons of herbal material into the mason jar and pour (almost) boiling water to the top. I cover the top but I typically don't close it up tight with the mason jar lid. I use a coaster or tea towel and then let it sit for 4 hours. Strain it and divide it into three cups for the day, or sip on it throughout the day. You can drink it hot (reheated) or cold.

TEA BLENDING

At some point the idea of blending herbs together to create your own tea blends will spark your curiosity. Perhaps it is because you want to blend a tea for sleep or a sore throat. This is one of my favorite things to do with students. Even those who say they have no palate for or experience in blending flavor combinations always seem to surprise themselves. Sure, you can stay the simple route and stick to using just one herb for your cups of tea, there is no fault in that. I, for one, drink straight chamomile almost every night. But, should you wish to get a little daring, try blending different herbs together and see how it comes out. This isn't without fail, by the way. I've blended plenty of herbs that ended up going right down the drain due to poor taste. Go into it as a learning experience and consider it a fun experiment.

One of the first things you need to consider is how certain herbs taste. This is similar to what many of us already do in the kitchen when adding spices to our foods. What is their flavor profile? If you have a bitter herb, consider balancing it with a sweet one, or a rooty earth flavor can be balanced with a little floral. You can learn flavor profiles by making a singular herb cup of tea and taking notes on what you think. Please keep in mind that everyone's thoughts on flavor are valid. Go with your gut, suss it out, and take good notes.

Another consideration with blending is the action of the herbs you are including. For example, if you want to make a tea to reduce a fever, it's best to not include spices such as cinnamon or cloves—these actually raise body temperature. When you understand the actions of what each herb does, you have the knowledge to create a tea blend with the intention to heal.

Blending is an art with a bit of science mixed in. You want it to produce the desired effect, but you also want it to taste good. There are three components of any good blend: healing potential, support of the body part affected, and flavor.

TEA BLENDING EXERCISE

Start with a healing intention, such as reducing fever or reducing digestive upset. Choose three herbs you want to include in your tea. For digestion, you might consider dogwood as your main herb because of its ability to support the entire digestive process, reducing bloating and gas. Then as a supporting herb you might consider elm because of its rich lignan content and ability to soothe the digestive tract. Now for flavor. In this example I would probably reach for peppermint, a natural digestive aid with great flavor. It also has a stimulant action, which means it will stimulate the other herbs, dogwood and elm, into action.

Next you'll need to play around with how much of each herb to put into the blend. The main herb, the one driving the healing intention, usually has the highest volume. Then the supporting herb, and then the flavor herb. Sometimes the supporting herb and the flavor herb are equal, but many times they have different ratios, depending on which herbs you use. Flavor herbs are usually very aromatic so they don't require much to add a lot of flavor. Keep it simple and use a ratio, say 2:1:0.5 for example. Start there and then you adjust to your preference. Another important consideration is that all blends should be made in small amounts until you get the hang of it. There is nothing worse than having to compost a pound of herbs you blended up because the flavor wasn't palatable. As for storage, I prefer glass mason jars. They keep the herbs fresh and free from oxygenation.

Exercise
Think of a tea blend you'd like to make. Some examples would be a tea for a head cold, sore throat, or one to drink after dinner to support digestion. Consider these three questions:

1. What is the focus of the tea, or the healing intention? What is this tea blend for?
2. What herb do you want to use as the main herb, the supporting herb and the flavor herb? Once you get more familiar with herbs and what they do in the body, this will get easier.
3. What should be your starting place for amounts? You can always add more of something but you can't take it away once the herbs have been blended together.

SYRUP

Roots, barks, and berries all make excellent syrups and can be made in the traditional stovetop way. The more delicate parts of plants, like leaves and flowers, can also be made into a syrup, but works better with an infusion method. See below for the directions for both.

Traditional Syrup Method
Great for tree berries, bark ,and roots such as hawthorn berries, elderberries, and poplar bark.

Specific amounts aren't given here as you will determine that by determining how much final product you wish to have. Instead I'll give you ratios. I like my syrups to be flavorful and bursting with medicinal potential, so I use the ratio of 1 cup of water to 1 tablespoon herb. The other ratio you need is the ratio of water to sugar, which is 1:1.

1 cup water : 1 tablespoon herb: 1 cup sugar
2 cups water: 2 tablespoon herb : 2 cups sugar
4 cups water : 4 tablespoon herb : 4 cups sugar
8 cups water : 8 tablespoon herb : 8 cups sugar

In this method you are using heat to dissolve the sugar as well as to reduce the liquid by half. This is what's known as a reduction. You are reducing the water to half of its original amount to yield a concentrated medicinal syrup.

Why use sugar? Honestly I asked this myself early on in my career and made syrups with various sweeteners including honey, maple syrup, and monk fruit. The reason sugar is used isn't to make the syrup sweet (although that is a great side effect) but because it's an effective preservative. Organic cane or turbinado sugar is a great preservative and I've ended up returning to it time after time when my syrups have gone off in short periods of time. Sugar alternatives can definitely be used, but I would suggest making small batches versus making and storing it until a time when it's needed, to reduce the risk of spoilage.

Place herbs in a thick-bottomed saucepan or smaller Dutch oven. Add water and bring to a boil. Boil it on medium or medium-low until the water is reduced by half. You don't want to boil it off too quickly, as that doesn't give the plant time to fully break down; similarly, too high of heat can damage the herb's medicinal properties.

After the mix has been reduced, strain the herbal compounds out once it is cool enough to handle safely. I like to set my strainer over a large glass measuring cup so I can accurately know how much sugar to add. Then return the liquid to the pot, measure out your sugar, add it and gently heat while stirring until sugar is completely dissolved.

If you want to ensure preservation for a long period of time, add food-grade citric acid, ½ teaspoon per cup of syrup.

Allow the syrup to cool and then store it in amber-colored bottles in a cool, dark place, or the refrigerator. Be sure to label the vials. Once opened, keep the syrup in the refrigerator and use it within 2 to 3 weeks.

INFUSION SYRUP

Great for blossoms like elderflower, lilac, and linden, and while they *are* all medicinal, they are perhaps more often considered a syrup to be used in the culinary world.

1 cup water : ½ cup herb : ¾ cup sugar : ¼ tsp. citric acid
2 cups water : 1 cup herb : 1½ cup sugar : ½ tsp. citric acid
4 cups water : 2 cup herb : 3 cups sugar : 1 tsp. citric acid
8 cups water : 4 cup herb : 6 cups sugar : 2 tsp. citric acid

In this method, first gently heat the water, sugar, and citric acid until dissolved. There is no need to boil with this method, so ensure you are using a gentle heat. Once dissolved, turn off the heat and let the mixture rest, covered, for 10 minutes.

In the meantime, trim and brush off all the debris from your herbs. I've found washing them reduces the flavor of the syrup, so I don't recommend that.

Fill up the appropriate-sized mason jar with the herbs and pour the sugar mixture over the top. Lay a kitchen towel over the opening and let it sit for 1 to 2 hours. Then move it to the refrigerator and let it steep for 4 days.

Strain the syrup with a very fine-mesh strainer or cheesecloth. Be sure to squeeze the herbs to liberate all of the syrup. Then bottle it up, label it, and enjoy.

HERBAL OIL

When a tree's medicinal parts are soluble in oil, their medicinal properties can be extracted into what is known as an herbal oil. This is *not* an essential oil. Essential oils are made through a distillation process using water and steam. Herbal oils are made by infusing plant material in oil using a heat source. The heat source can even be the sun, as long as it is hot enough, or the oven.

Oil types to consider:
Olive, grapeseed oil, apricot, castor, jojoba, or almond oil.

Sun Method
Fill a mason jar with freshly harvested tree material, such a birch bark. You want the jar to be packed with the bark, but not so tightly that oil can't seep down in between the pieces. Next, simply pour the oil over the bark, to the top of the jar. Cover the jar with cheesecloth and a rubber band to hold it in place.

Set in a very warm and sunny place. The cheesecloth allows for any water in the bark to evaporate and reduces the risk of contaminating the oil. The outside temperatures must reach mid-80s F, or above, for this process to be successful.

Remove the cheesecloth every 4 or 5 days to evaluate and give a stir. Be sure to smell it also to ensure everything is on track. The alternative to stirring is to remove the cheesecloth and put on a mason jar lid and give it a shake. Then remove it and put the cheesecloth back on.

Infuse the oil for 2 to 3 weeks and then strain with a fine-mesh strainer and/or cheesecloth, ensuring you are squeezing all of the oil from the herb.

Store in a dark-colored container in a cool, dark place. Be sure to label it with name and date of production.

Oven Method
The oven method is great when you need to make an herbal oil in the winter, such as with poplar buds. I suggest dedicating one of your old glass baking dishes to your herbal endeavors because getting it completely clean can be challenging. Residue from resins and such is common but because they are antimicrobial/antibacterial.

Line the bottom of your baking dish with your herb of choice and then pour the oil over the top, filling it until you see 1 to 2 inches of oil below the herb. Give it a good stir to saturate the herb; it will begin to sink to the bottom of the pan.

Turn the oven to 150°F and "bake" the oil for 4 to 6 hours. I like to check on it every hour, giving it a stir. This probably isn't necessary, but being part of the process is enjoyable. The best part is the lovely aroma that begins to fill the house. Be sure to let it cool before you strain the oil with a fine-mesh strainer and/or cheesecloth, ensuring you squeeze all of the oil from the herb.

Store the oil in a dark-colored container in a cool, dark place; be sure to label and date it.

SALVE, MUSCLE RUB, BALM

Now that you know how to make herbal oil, you are ready to make an herbal salve. Herbal oils and salves are also used as the base to make body butters, muscle rubs, and balms. Salves are the old-fashioned term for a spreadable medicine that is often put on cuts, burns, and wounds.

Traditionally, lard was used to make the balm thicker but today the most common base is beeswax. There are also vegan waxes available. As a beekeeper, I always have excess wax around from cleaning hives, so that is what I use.

3 milliliters herbal oil : 1 milliliter melted beeswax
300 milliliters herbal oil : 100 milliliters melted beeswax

Gently heat your herbal oil and add the beeswax, stirring with a metal spoon until completely dissolved.

Immediately pour it into your tins, jars, or container of choice and allow it to cool completely before putting the lid on top. If you put the lid on while it is still cooling you'll get condensation on top of the salve and a concave dip in the center of the salve.

The Tried-and-True Spoon Test
If you aren't sure if you've added enough or too much beeswax, try the spoon test. Using a metal spoon, scoop up some of the salve mixture and set the spoon on a piece of wax paper in the refrigerator for 5 to 8 minutes. Pull it from the fridge and test the hardness of salve on the spoon. Is it too soft? Add more beeswax. If it is too hard, add more herbal oil.

POULTICE

A poultice is a paste or soft moist mass of plant material with healing properties. They are quick and easy to apply and often yield fast results. Taking a leaf with known astringent properties, chewing it up in your mouth and then placing it over a wound can be imperative at times when out in the wilderness. At home, we can use a mortar and pestle with a bit of warm water to make a macerated paste and then apply it as needed. I often spread the poultice on the affected/wounded area, cover it with a piece of medical gauze, and tape it down to hold it in place.

In a mortar and pestle grind and macerate 4 to 6 leaves of choice. Transfer this to a small mixing bowl and add teaspoons of hot water until a thick paste forms. You don't want to add the water to the mortar because they are often made of porous material and best kept dry. Apply the poultice to the intended area and leave on for 30 minutes or overnight if wrapped well.

Poultices are great for bug bites, sprains, strains, colds, sinus issues, wounds, cuts, headaches, relaxing, and so much more.

FOMENTATION

A fomentation is similar to a poultice, but instead of applying the plant material directly to the skin, you are making a very steep herbal infusion, soaking a cloth in that infusion and then wrapping the affected area.

Set the kettle to boil and put 1 cup of herbs into a large stockpot. Add three cups of hot water, cover and let steep for 30 minutes. Remove the cover to allow steam to escape. Once it is cool enough to touch, soak a cotton cloth or towel in the tea. Wring out the excess and then wrap the area. You can cover it with another towel or plastic wrap to hold it in place if necessary.

This is great for broken bones, rashes, sore throats, sprains, and strains.

CAPSULES

A popular choice for obvious reasons, capsules are convenient as there is no taste and they are great for traveling.

If you'd like to experiment making capsules, I recommend you invest in a personal capsule maker, something like the Cap.M.Quik or the Capsule Machine. These handy tools make it easy to make homemade capsules. But if you prefer to do it by hand, you certainly can.

You'll need to grind your herbs in a nut, seed, or herb grinder until a very fine powder, then put it into a bowl.

For the capsule tools, you'll start by pulling apart the number of empty capsules you want to make. Put the tops in a bowl and line the bottom tray with the bottom capsule. Next pour the powder over the tray and use the spreading tool to fill up all the capsules. Then you'll put the tops on and voilà, you've got capsules.

Otherwise, by hand, you can pull apart one capsule at a time and, holding either end in either hand, dip each into the bowl of powder and then push the capsule halves together. It's a bit more messy but easy to do.

TINCTURES

Herbal-based tinctures are an old folk remedy where the plant material is macerated (soaked in liquid) to pull the medicinal properties out of the plant and into the liquid. The traditional solvent, the liquid used to macerate, is alcohol. Alcohol is primarily used because it can easily break down the plant parts and often pulls more medicinal constituents out than water and/or oil. The other advantage of an alcohol-based medicine is that it bypasses the digestive tract. Tinctures are absorbed sublingually, which means they immediately enter the bloodstream when taken. This is very handy when you need your medicine to work quickly.

The two types of tincture production are maceration and percolation. And then you can make a maceration tincture in two different ways. The two ways are the folk method, which I'll describe below, and the standardized method. The standardized method is great for when you want to duplicate exact results or you wish to control the solvent range. It is also required for commercial production. This method can be used by anyone, but for the home herbalists, the folk method works great and is much simpler. If you want to learn about percolations and/or the standardized method, check out my book *The Herbal Apothecary* for step-by-step instructions.

Folk Method
I've made tinctures in all sorts of ways and quite honestly, the folk method is my favorite way. So many of our modern ways have replaced the older traditions, but some things just don't need to be reinvented. You can use fresh or dried tree parts to make tinctures, but when you use the fresh parts there is something magical in seeing the colors change and catching the scents as it macerates.

Fresh vol. 1 herb : 2 alcohol
Dried vol. 1 herb : 4-5 alcohol

Glass mason jars work best for making tinctures and having the measuring marks on the side of the jar makes it easier to identify the ratios. If you have a 16-oz. jar and want to make a fresh tincture, fill it up halfway with fresh plant material. Be sure to pack it somewhat but not too tight. Don't stress—there is no wrong way here; you'll still wind up with some medicine even if the ratio isn't perfect.

With fresh plant material you'll need to use a slightly higher percentage of alcohol because you need to account for the water still in the plant. I typically use a diluted cane alcohol at 60-75%. Fill to the top of the jar and tightly close. Be sure to label the name and part of the plant being macerated, the day's date you processed it, and a date 3 to 4 weeks in the future. The future date is the day you'll be straining and pouring this into storage bottles. Store the tincture in a dark, cool space but make sure it is accessible because daily agitation of the jar is necessary. Every day, pull out the jar and give it a good shake for 60 seconds. At the end of 3 to 4 weeks, strain. Again, there is no hard-and-fast rule here. Some herbalists will say 2 weeks is plenty but one thing we seem to all agree on is that after 4 weeks, there is nothing more to extract from the plant. Macerating it longer does not produce a stronger tincture.

When you strain it, be sure to really squeeze all of the plant material to collect every last drop. If you prefer not to do it by hand, there are herbal tincture presses available to purchase. Pour it into storage bottles and keep in a cool, dark place. Tightly sealed and unopened, tinctures can be stored forever. While the FDA will put a number on it of 5 to 10 years, as long as it is stored properly, what can go bad if it is preserved in alcohol? But if you've opened it and it has been exposed to oxygen, then yes, after a couple of years it is best to dispose of it and start fresh.

Dried Herbs
Making a tincture with the folk method for dried herbs is the exact same process but with two considerable differences. One is the herb-to-alcohol ratio. Most herbals will recommend a 1:5 ratio, and most of the time I agree. But sometimes, I switch to a 1:4 ratio with certain blends. I mention this only because if you want to try it, or feel intuitively that it should be a bit stronger of a tincture, then go for it. The other difference is the alcohol percentage. The dried material has all of the water evaporated out of it and therefore doesn't need a high alcohol percentage. If too high, it can burn the plant material and destroy the medicinal properties. Using a 80- to 100-proof vodka is perfect for dried folk method tinctures.

Last note: I am all about flavor when I make tinctures. I really don't like tinctures that taste like lighter fluid and to be honest, there is no need for that. One thing to remember is that when you go to buy vodka at the liquor store, the higher it sits on the shelf, the better the quality. If you choose a bottom-shelf brand, be prepared to breathe fire.

Some tree parts can be macerated in apple cider vinegar or vegetable glycerin in place of alcohol. The key here is to know which ones. Be sure to do your research or check out the list in *The Herbal Apothecary*.

A little tip: Leave a little room in your tinctures and add a touch of vegetable glycerin and/or apple cider vinegar. Both of these soften the alcohol flavor and can provide a more pleasurable taste.

HERBAL BATHS AND STEAMS

Using herbs in baths and steams was once a pivotal component to nature healing. In our modern era we tend to believe that baths take too long, which is a bit of an oxymoron because that is precisely the point! We should slow down, especially when we aren't well.

A full bath is when your entire body is in the bath and there are herbs infused in the bath water.

A half bath is usually in a Japanese-style tub, where you are only submerged from the navel down.

A sitz bath is a bath performed in a smaller tub that only submerges your bum, hips, and lower belly.

An eye bath is helpful with eye infections, sore eyes, or hayfever.

A footbath is when just the feet are submerged up to the ankles and is great for sore feet, infections, rashes, yeast, cuts, or wounds.

A vapor bath (steam) is utilized when the head is full of congestion and mucous, or to help clear the skin of rash, infection, or acne.

Medicinal Trees and Recipes

Acacia

Acacia spp., Valchellia tortilis subsp. raddiana, Acacia senegal (Senegalia greggii), Valchellia nilotica subsp. tomentosa, Vachellia nilotica

Family: Fabaceae
Parts used: bark, gum, leaves, seeds
Medicinal actions: astringent, demulcent, emollient
Native geography: tropical and subtropical regions around the world, especially Australia and Africa; certain species native to southwestern US and northern Mexico

I was on a four-month sabbatical, designed to help me get my bearings in preparation for the next phase of my life. I'd lately also been having dreams about acacia trees. If you close your eyes and think of a picturesque, twisted tree with a flat canopy in the middle of a desert, it is most likely an acacia. They've always fascinated me with their tenacity. Their feathery compound leaves create a dreamlike canopy over the desert floor. I'd personify them by saying they look like they must be lonely, as they often appear growing alone, with a backdrop of an expansive, beautiful horizon. The intermittent shade they produce, though, attracts people and animals alike throughout the day. Until this trip, I'd only seen them in books and on TV. Graduate school took six years, and at the same time I opened a medicinal herb shop. My "on" switch had been perpetually in high gear, and I knew I needed to turn it off for a minute to see if my future was heading in the direction I wanted it to be going. So I made a plan to visit places I'd always dreamed of, ending with Egypt and a trip up Mt. Sinai. Acacia trees grow wild there.

People have always thought I am crazy for traveling alone, but I quite enjoy it. Don't get me wrong, I love traveling with people too, but there is an unfurling of self that happens when I am alone. I'm more aware of myself and my surroundings. My autopilot for fulfilling roles I play at home no longer takes over, because everything is new and different. My perception becomes keen, like a hawk watching all from above. When these aspects of myself show up, I become more present and comfortable with exploring. Without regimented schedules, routines, and deadlines I am able to think about the choices I'm making—and change course as needed.

I began the journey to Mt. Sinai at one in the morning. I won't sugarcoat it, there are times when solo traveling requires a deep stretch of self to assess the situations you find yourself in. My male driver showed up in a black SUV with dark tinted windows in the middle of the night and opened the door for me. I took a deep breath, told myself that I had selected trustworthy people to make these arrangements for me, and got in. We drove on sand highways through the desert. I could just barely make out the rising and falling of dunes around us. Once we arrived, I stepped out of the car and into quite a different scene. One that was energetic, akin to a lively dusk scene at a county fair.

I looked around and saw people and camels, moving mostly in small groups preparing for the trek up the mountain. Despite the darkness, my driver quickly found my guide. He was a friendly, and very round, bedouin man. For an instant I worried about his physical state; could he really guide me up this mountain? But, after brief introductions, off we went. We walked over to the trailhead, then he asked me to wait a few minutes and quickly skittered away. Maybe he needed one last biobreak before heading up? This is what I told myself in attempt to quiet the panicked thought that I'd just been abandoned. As I scanned around for him, I pressed my hand against a tree trunk. I looked up, and saw that this tree was spread out like an umbrella

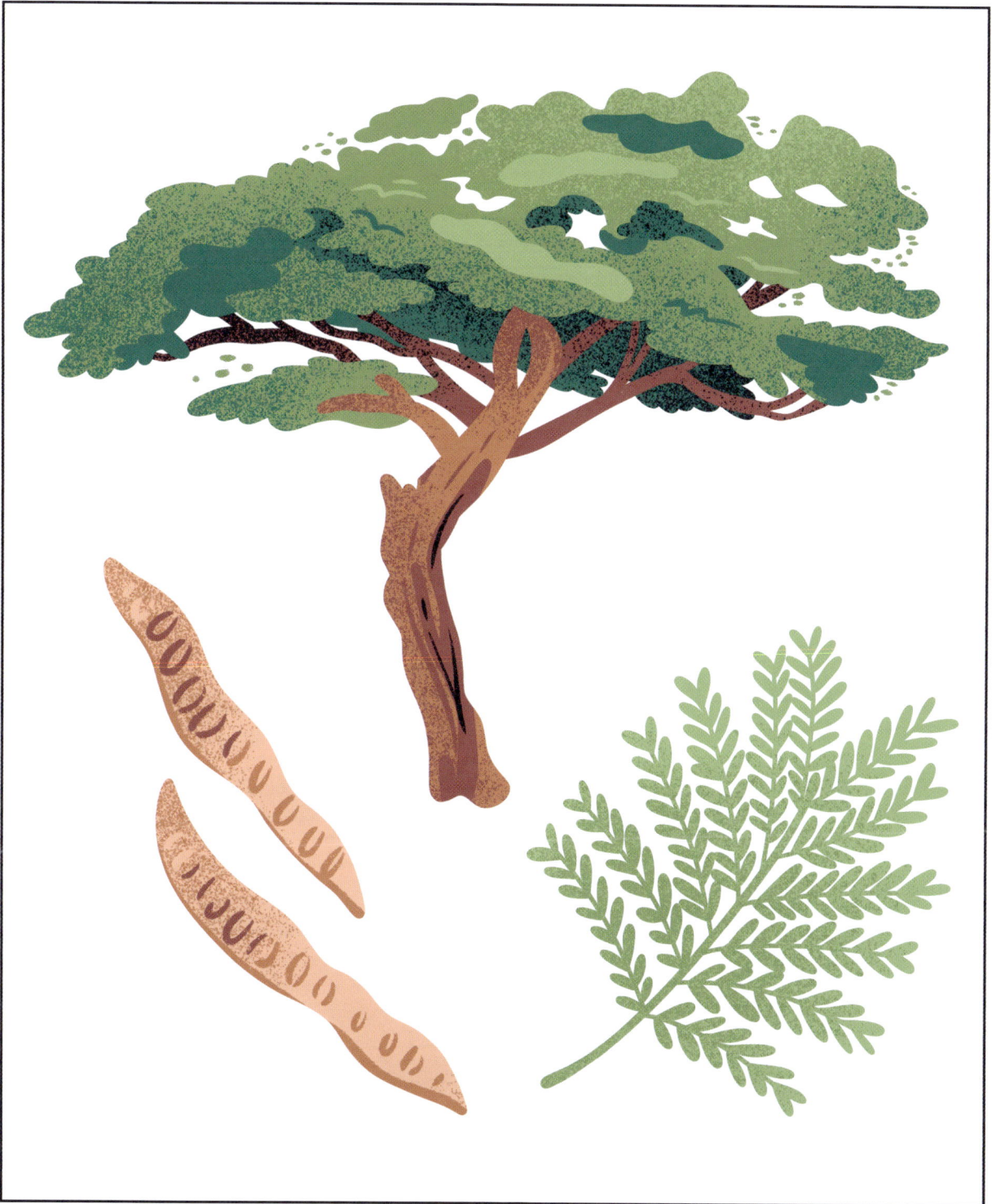

USDA hardiness zones: 9 to 11

Water: water regularly during first season after planting, then acacia becomes extremely drought tolerant

Light requirement: full sun

Soil: Fertile, well-drained soil with a slightly acidic pH

Temperature: intolerant of freezing

Wildlife notes: a rare foraging site for some bat species, ants have a healthy mutualistic relationship with the tree

Pollinator friendly: all pollinators are drawn to this tree for its flowers and nectar, including butterflies

Pests: prone to fungus, mildew, comma moths; saplings are prone to damp-off

and had spiny thorns. Tears sprang to my eyes. Here was the very tree, supporting me now, that I'd been feeling a subconscious connection to (my entire life). Just as my emotions were getting the best of me, my guide returned—with a camel. A tall coffee-with-cream-colored animal with beautifully braided reins clopped up to the acacia, happy to take a nibble. When I explained I preferred to walk, as so many had before me, the guide tied him to the tree.

As with most treks, first exertion elicits a certain excitement, then I tend to fall into a sort of meditative state as I move step by step. I could see my feet, placed them one in front of the other in time to the rhythmic swaying of my guide's thobe (his long gown). I'd never climbed at night before, and it felt as if I were climbing toward the stars. We rarely saw anyone else along the narrow trail, and when we did only hushed greetings and exchanges were made as we passed. The stars were 10 million strong, and I counted over a dozen shooting stars as we zigzagged back and forth along the path.

Suddenly, on a little plateau, we came to a teahouse. It was simple, constructed of wood and sheepskins and perched on an outcrop of rock. The scent of tea wafted in the air. The smell of all three created a unique aroma that, like a tattoo, marked this memory onto my brain. The tea was unfortunately unremarkable but the heat it injected into my chilled body was just what I needed. My guide and I, with several others, huddled around a small fire in silence as we contemplated the next part of the hike.

We climbed higher, foot by foot. After three hours, we reached what seemed like another little plateau. My guide stopped, went over to a pile of bed mats that had manifested out of the darkness, grabbed two, and started turning in circles, looking for a place to lay

them on the ground. When he found what he deemed a good spot, he announced that we were "here." Here? Because of the darkness (no flashlights), I was completely disoriented. He lay down on his mat and told me to do the same. He said that because I was a fast walker, we had time to rest for a bit. Rest? I didn't want to—my mind was overstimulated by the trek (and quite possibly, the tea). But I did as told and cuddled down into the mat and wool blanket. It was a restless rest, my active mind and tired body at odds.

After about an hour, I noticed peaks of color beginning to lighten up the horizon. I sat up a few times to watch the navy darkness being slowly replaced with pinks and reds, then I'd lie back down for a few moments. But once the cotton-candy sky turned into streaks of orange and yellow, I felt my energy beginning to boil over. I never tire of sunrises. Each one is magical, and I always notice slight differences in the shades, clouds, or bursts of light, and Mt. Sinai felt particularly special. My guide asked me why I was taking so many pictures. I just smiled and watched. The sky's color intensified and brightened, and the increasing amount of joy in my chest kept pace.

As the day dawned, I realized my guide had perched us on the edge of a plateau. Nothing but mountains and sky extended on a horizon in front of me. And right as the sun crested over the mountainous horizon, the pinnacle of any sunrise, I suddenly heard an incredible chorus of whoops and hollers and exclamations. I knew I had been climbing toward the heavens on one of humanity's most sacred sites, so for a moment I honestly thought I was hallucinating the sounds of angels. As I slowly turned to look behind me to see who else was there, I realized there were hundreds of fellow trekkers with me on that plateau; all had made the same pilgrimage to reach the summit in time for this moment, and we shared an instant connection. And then I saw a glorious acacia tree lit up in pure, white light.

———————

Acacias have been mentioned by various cultures and religions across human history, since it survives so well in desert and arid landscapes. Acacia trees add visual interest to any area with their twisted trunks and horizontal, umbrella-like canopies. Growing up to 6 meters (19.5 feet) tall, it has a curious growth pattern. Typically when water is scarce, the taproots burrow deep into the earth, which in turn causes the tree to grow large quickly. It is known to survive for months through severe droughts. The leaves are pinnately compound, 3.5–8 centimeters (1.4–3 inches) long, creating welcome shade on hot afternoons. It bears prickly branches armed with three-hooked thorns up to 7 millimeters (0.3 inches) long that emerge just below nodes on branches.

The trees flower at various times depending on zone and species, and are either white or yellow. The flowers grow in axillary spikes, appearing before the leaves. They are almost fuzzy looking from a distance and produce a very pleasant scent. The seed pods, which can grow up to 9 centimeters (3.5 inches), are vibrant green before slowly drying to a paper-thin, crispy brown shell.

Acacia gum is harvested in the dry season. Much like tapping maple syrup, an incision is made on the trunk (this does not permanently damage the tree). Within several weeks, gum seeps into the incisions, then dries partially upon exposure to air and forms a nodule. Every two to four weeks, these nodules can be harvested and dried completely in the sun. This resinous compound is then stored in airtight containers, in a cool and dark place. As long as it has been dried properly, gum resin can be stored for up to three years. Modern herbalists often begin using an herb in a trial-and-error way to gain experience with our own eyes as to what works for a given injury or pathology. But with acacia, we can draw on a centuries-long tradition of use for drying mucosal membranes, in reducing inflammatory diarrhea and respiratory disease.

———————

Acacia is reported to have antibacterial effects against pathogenic microorganisms such as *Mycobacterium tuberculosis*, *Pseudomonas aeruginosa*, *Escherichia coli* and *Staphylococcus aureus*. *A. nilotica* showed high antimicrobial potential against *S. aureus*, *E. coli*, *Salmonella typhi* and *Klebsiella pneumoniae* in a comparative antimicrobial study among acacia species. This helps us better understand its success in patients with chronic diarrhea in the nineteenth century when many other astringent herbal treatments failed. And with infectious lung diseases that never seem to improve. It is also used on skin burns, particularly those at risk of infection, but also on any type of skin inflammation that is in need of soothing. I typically reach for acacia when there is an infectious or inflamed mucous membrane in the alimentary (mouth to anus), respiratory, or urinary canals. It is particularly helpful against bacterial infection but also at soothing inflammation and pain. Its demulcent nature coats and calms down irritated tissues and its astringency factor helps absorb excess fluid.

Acacia Recipes

INDICATIONS

- Asthma
- Breastfeeding pain, apply topically
- Diarrhea
- Dysentery
- Gum irritation and disease
- High cholesterol
- Kidney and bladder infection, pain
- Lung bacterial infection, pneumonia, tuberculosis, bronchitis
- Skin burns, inflammation, irritations

HERBAL TOOTH POWDER

Acacia makes a great powdered toothpaste that is nonabrasive and cleans plaque efficiently.

Items needed:
Grafting and/or drawing knife
Collecting bowl
Acacia gum or powder
Mortar and pestle
Glass storage container

Collect acacia gum from a tree at least five years old. Make several rectangular incisions in the stem and/or branches of the tree, approximately 1–2 inches by 3–4 inches, then strip this area of bark. This does not damage the tree, but encourages the tree to produce gum to cover the incision, like a natural bandage covering a wound. Gum droplets will seep out and protrude like a balloon. Some droplets will be small, while others puff to the size of a baseball. Depending on the weather, let them seep for 3 to 8 weeks. Once exposed to the air and sunlight, the gum will dry and harden into resinlike "tears" that can be manually gathered into a bowl.

After the resin has been collected, let it rest for a day or two to dry fully. Then use a mortar and pestle to grind it into a fine powder, and store in a glass container.

If you haven't used tooth powder before, it can take a minute to get used to how it feels, but the transition is relatively easy from commercial paste. Wet your toothbrush, then dip the bristles into the herbal powder or sprinkle it on. Brush for two minutes and rinse.

RAAB AYURVEDIC IMMUNITY BEVERAGE

The sap of acacia trees has been used in traditional Indian cooking and medicine for centuries. This traditional ayurvedic drink improves digestion, supports women postpartum, and fights off colds.

Items needed:
Heavy-bottom pan
Cooking spoon
Plate lined with a paper towel
Small bowl or tea mug

Ingredients:
1 tbsp. clarified butter or ghee
1½ tbsp. acacia gum
1½ cups water, milk, or plant-based milk
2 tbsp. unrefined cane sugar
½ tsp. ground cardamom
½ tsp. ground dry ginger
¼ tsp. ground turmeric
¼ tsp. ground cloves
1/16 tsp. ground cayenne
1 tbsp. desiccated coconut
1 tsp. almond powder
     (from 4-5 ground almonds)
4 slivered almonds

Add ghee or butter to a heavy-bottomed pan on medium heat until melted. Add the acacia gum, stirring often. After it puffs up and fries, use a slotted spoon to scoop it out and set it on a paper-towel-lined plate. Allow to fully cool, then grind into a powder. (If you want to shorten the process, purchase powdered acacia and start at the next step.)

Add the powder back to the pan along with the rest of the ingredients, stirring constantly on low to medium heat. Bring to a boil. Once the sugar is completely dissolved, pour into a mug and top with slivered almonds.

Drink on cold winter mornings to warm up and start the day boosted against colds and flus.

Ash

Fraxinus americana,
Fraxinus excelsior

Family: Oleaceae
Parts used: leaves,
bark, fruit
Medicinal actions:
alterative, astringent,
anti-inflammatory,
anti-microbial, febrifuge,
laxative
Native geography:
eastern North America;
Europe and the Caucasus, Turkey, Iran

**Do not confuse with
prickly ash, bitter ash,
or mountain ash*

They called it lightning snow. It was October in Lincoln, Nebraska, and we'd barely turned the corner into fall when we had a crazy snowstorm. Feet upon feet of snow fell, mixed with rain and ice—and lightning. It was the type of storm where I held fear and fascination close to my chest. I noticed that my breaths were coming short and sharp. My brain could not make sense of it, because lightning and snow aren't supposed to happen at the same time.

In the front yard of our shotgun bungalow stood the perfect ash tree. It had most likely been planted there to shade the house, because ash trees are extremely fast-growing, and this one had been well maintained. It leafed out so well in the summer that our home was at least five degrees cooler on hot days. Whoever had lived there before us cut the lower branches and trimmed the outer ones to give it the perfect cartoonish tree shape, all proportionally round and bushy. There was a swing there, but since we didn't have kids and we weren't anywhere near that stage in our lives, we had changed it out for a bird feeder.

Because the news loves to sensationalize any type of snowstorm, we had plenty of warning it was coming. In Nebraska we typically didn't worry too much about severe weather; we simply moved through life aware of it. In the spring, tornado sirens often sent us to the basement. Flash floods in the summer made for wild car rides. With my brother, sister, and I squished in the backseat we'd often hear our parents whispering up front, "Do you think the car can make it?" And

winter simply meant ice and snow. It rarely mattered to our school or our boss if snow was falling. Warming up the car and scraping the windshield was just a part of a Nebraskan's life. Fall, though, was the one season where weather was calm. It was the one season we had off. Maybe that is why the news station decided to amplify the warnings about the possible intensity of this storm. But still, even as the snow began to fall, none of us thought much about it. After all, we were used to our cars sliding all over the road on the way home from work. Once settled at home, my boyfriend and I watched it from the safety of our screened-in porch. Tucked underneath blankets on an old lumpy couch, we watched the water fall from the sky, oscillating from rain to snow to ice. We were in awe at this unexpected event suddenly taking the main stage of our lives. We even ran outside from time to time to see how the different types of precipitation felt on our hands and faces. Yes, the news had told us it was coming, but it is different once it all begins out of season.

As dusk fell, we talked in the darkness, taking turns making hot drinks, and sometimes just sitting quietly. At some point in the middle of the night, long after we'd gone to bed, we awoke to the worst sound I think I have ever heard. It sounded like our bedroom was being split right in two. A slow, deep, and so-so-loud cracking that seemed to surround us entirely. I thought Godzilla might be standing outside, ripping the roof off. We could barely hear each other as we scrambled from our bedroom to the living room. Then, all at once, the noise stopped. Silence. I'd

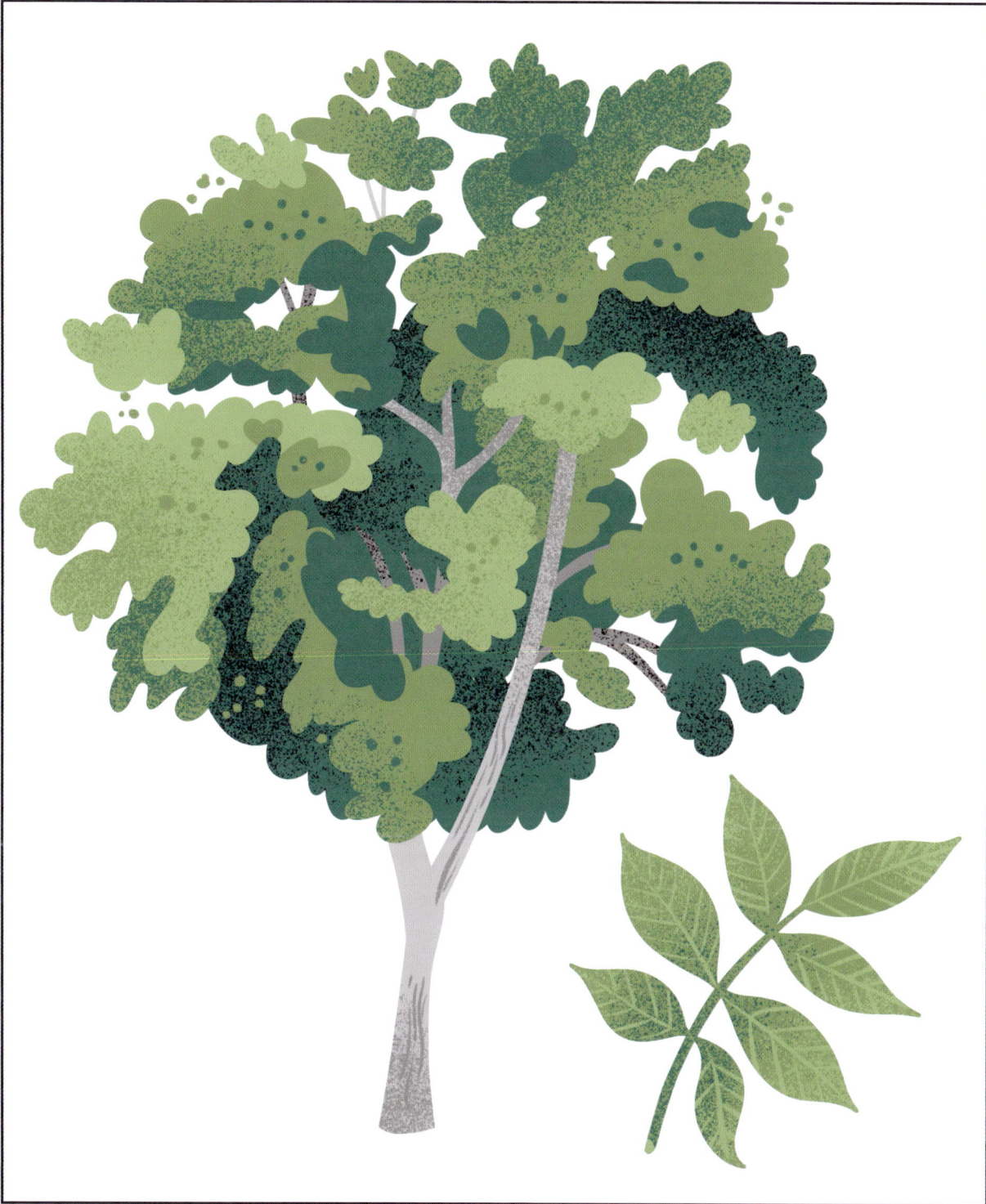

never heard such utter silence. At some point, I noticed that we were panting. Had our roof collapsed? Did someone drive into the side of the house? It felt like slow motion leapt into fast-forward as we crept around, looking for the cause of the noise. Seeing nothing, we turned to the front door and walked out onto the screen porch.

There was snow everywhere, almost three feet covering every inch of everything. And on top of the snow was a sheet of solid ice two inches thick. It glistened as we shined a flashlight around. Looking into the front yard, we saw that our prized ash tree had split from top to button, almost perfectly in half. The right half of the tree laid across our yard and driveway, having just missed my car by inches. The left half of the tree still stood perfectly erect, its branches glistening from the ice reflected in the yellow glow of the streetlight. And hanging from the lowest branch, as if nothing had happened at all, was the frozen bird feeder, unmoving.

The branches from the right half of the ash tree ended up providing an abundant harvest of medicinal bark, but we realized that the cambium on the trunk was still intact, so we decided to graft the felled portion back onto the standing tree. I honestly never expected it to work, but within a year it wove itself back together and continued to grow.

Follow the white-tailed deer and you'll most likely be led to an ash tree before long. It is loved by many forest animals including beavers, porcupines, rabbits, squirrels, and many varieties of birds, as it provides endless resources in terms of both food and nesting materials. Ash trees are occasionally mentioned in older Western herbal texts, but they are more commonly recognized as a valuable

medicine source in Chinese medicine and by American Indian tribes from the East Coast of North America. I typically reserve ash for simple remedies including the relief of constipation when it's accompanied with bloating, fever, and skin issues like pruritus (itchiness). A little medicinal-strength tea usually clears up these complaints.

There are some interesting accounts of ash working to reduce the size of enlarged organs, particularly the uterus and spleen. It would be interesting to try after childbirth to aid the uterus in returning to pre-pregnancy size. Research has shown high antioxidant properties in ash leaves, due to the presence of flavonoid glycosides. The bark shows strong antimicrobial properties. Other research has identified anticancer, anti-inflammatory, neuroprotective, antianginal, and antihypertensive effects.

In Chinese medicine ash is referred to by its pin yin name, Qin Pi. If you've not explored Chinese medicine as a healing modality, I strongly encourage it. Understanding your own body through a traditional medicine philosophy can only complement modern medicine techniques. This tradition uses ash to support the liver, gallbladder, stomach, and large intestine, particularly when there is "dampness" in the body. An easy way to understand "dampness" in Chinese medicine is when there is excess water that creates an imbalance and inhibits energy circulation. Think of it like a bog in your body.

Ash trees grow as much as 0.3 to 0.6 meters (1 to 2 feet) per year, so they can quickly fill in landscapes. Ash is very adaptable—in other words, forgiving—which is great for beginner gardeners. While it will grow without requiring too much attention, it thrives in moist, deep, well-drained soils and full sun. Young saplings are easily transplanted. They will often grow up to 12 meters (40 feet) before extending new branches, then begin to branch outward.

Ash leaves are deciduous, opposite, pinnately compound and approximately 20 to 38 centimeters (8 to 15 inches) long. Ash trees are dioecious, meaning that male and female flowers typically grow on different trees. But sometimes male flowers will emerge on one branch and female flowers on another. The flowers, which come in April and May, are delicate and very small. They range from green to a deep purple, are in clusters near the branch tips and often have a fragrant scent.

The bark is commonly light gray, but it can vary a bit to a yellow-brown. Young trees have smooth, soft-feeling bark; it turns rough and deeply furrowed with age. Some say it looks like a pulled net pattern running up and down the trunk.

The Natural Resources Conservation Service of the US Agriculture department has identified that white ash is sensitive to ozone, sulfur dioxide, nitrous oxides, and associated acid deposition. When high levels of these gases are in the environment, it causes the appearance of necrotic lesions on the leaves. This, along with the emerald ash borer, have caused ash decline over the last several decades.

The leaves are best harvested in mid-to-late spring, in the early morning hours. After drying them, you can cut them up for tea, or grind them into a powder for storage. The inner bark is harvested most often in late winter. To gather the inner bark, take long vertical strips from the trunk, not horizontal. Gather from branches and fallen limbs if possible, and above all avoid girdling the tree with scars.

Ash Recipes

INDICATIONS

- Arthritis
- Constipation due to water retention
- Dandruff
- Digestive tonic
- Fever
- Prolapse of uterus and bladder
- Rheumatism
- Snake and insect bites
- Splenomegaly

May lower blood glucose levels and/or blood pressure. If currently on medications for either of these, be sure to closely monitor and consult your practitioner.

HAIR RINSE

The Greeks, Romans, and ancient Javanese all used rinses to nourish and moisturize hair. They are also great to reduce scalp dandruff and eczema and can be used to treat lice. Ash hair rinse leaves the hair shiny and strong, down to the follicles.

Items needed:
Stockpot
Cooking spoon
Strainer
Glass measuring cup with pour spout
Funnel
16-oz. plastic storage bottle with squirt top

Ingredients:
18 oz. water
1 oz. American ash bark
Rosemary essential oil

Put the water in the pot and bring it to a boil. Add the ash bark and give it a stir. Let it boil gently for 5 minutes, then turn off the heat and cover. Let sit until completely cooled.

Strain into the measuring cup and then, using the funnel, pour into the storage bottle.

Add 20 to 30 drops of the rosemary essential oil, depending on scent preference.

It's best to apply a hair rinse after a regular wash and conditioning. Squirt it onto the head and massage it in gently to ensure it gets from the top to the bottom of every strand of hair. Leave it on for at least one minute and then rinse, preferably with cool water.

PICKLED ASH KEYS

As a fan of the slow food movement, I like making things that take time. Fermented foods such as kimchi and sauerkraut are often in my crock, doing what they do until they are ready to be eaten. Pickled ash seeds have a slightly spicy flavor that some have compared to cardamom, but the pickled keys taste of walnuts. They're often eaten throughout Europe and Asia. Harvest the keys as they are just forming, before the seed begins to grow inside. An easy way to check is to hold them up to the light to determine the seeds' progress.

Items needed:
Stockpot
Strainer
Double boiler
Small mixing bowl
Muslin cloth
Glass measuring cup with pour spout
2 8-oz. canning jars and lids

Ingredients:
2 cups of ash keys, no stalks
2 tbsp. brown sugar
1 tsp. ground cloves
1 tsp. ground cinnamon
4 juniper berries
4 bay leaves
8 peppercorns
1 tsp. allspice
½ tsp. ground ginger
1 tsp. salt
2 cups apple cider vinegar, or 1½ cup apple cider
    and ½ cup of flowering currant cider

Rinse the ash keys in cold water in the sink, then add them to your stockpot and cover with water by 4 or 5 inches. Bring to a boil, then lower heat and simmer, uncovered, for 5 minutes. Strain. Fill the stockpot again with fresh water and repeat the boil/simmering process. Then strain again.

Lay keys on clean kitchen towels and gently pat off excess water.

Pack the keys into the jars, allowing one inch of space at the top of the jar. You want the jar to be full, but not compacted.

Mix all of the spices, salt, and sugar together in a bowl and add the vinegar (and cider if using).

Dump the contents of the bowl into the top of the double boiler, and add water to the lower pot.

Bring up to a gentle boil and simmer for 5 minutes. Turn off the heat and let the liquid cool completely.

Strain the spice/vinegar mixture through a muslin-lined strainer into a glass measuring cup with a pour spout.

Pour the strained liquid over the ash keys in the jars. Close tightly with a lid and give them a gentle shake.

Store in a cool, dry place for 3 months to allow the keys to pickle.

Banyan

Ficus benghalensis

Family: Moraceae
Parts used: bark, leaves, roots, and fruit
Medicinal actions: anti-inflammatory, antimicrobial, antioxidant, antispasmodic, astringent, demulcent, vulnerary
Native geography: Asia, from India through Myanmar, Thailand, Southeast Asia, southern China, and Malaysia

It was reported in December of 2023 that 60 percent of the famous and beloved banyan tree in Lahaina, on the Hawaiian island of Maui, was showing new green growth. When I heard this news, I exhaled a breath I didn't even know I'd been holding. I'd prayed for that tree, as had thousands of others, when wildfire devastated the city in August, earlier that same year—the result of downed powerlines. This sacred banyan had played a role in the life of Lahaina for 150 years, acting as a meeting spot where locals and tourists came together in the recognized space of community.

I'd sat under that tree, in the company of dozens of strangers, during my second visit to Hawaii; it was the perfect place to take a break from the heat, a break from life. Banyans have wide and low-reaching branches that arch out in every direction like arms grasping for something to hug. Prop roots hang down from the branches, thick like ropes that make you want to grab one and swing like a monkey. Much to any kid's dismay, climbing this nest of outstretched branches is discouraged. Some kids were anyway the day I was there, squawking and screaming; it was as if the ones in the tree and the others running around below would, for moments at a time, claim the tree as their own. As I sat there, I contemplated whether the tree felt joy from the attention of all of these children. If it could absorb and radiate back out the love it perhaps felt?

When I was eight years old, my grandma had vacationed here. At the time it had seemed like an exciting and exotic place for her to travel. Like any good grandma, she returned with a suitcase full of trinkets and souvenirs—including two beach towels for my sister and me. I didn't really like mine, but the one my sister nabbed was something I secretly coveted for decades. It featured a graphic that's the classic white person's vision of Hawaii: blue waves, sunset over the ocean, and a hula dancer with jet black hair in a traditional grass skirt. As a naive child living in a landlocked state, it captured my heart and mind and I wanted every inch of that tropical land.

It wasn't until I'd been living in the Pacific Northwest for nine years that I made my first voyage over to the islands. I had been craving lush coastlines, sandy beaches, and blue waters. A last-minute decision and a maxed-out credit card landed me smack in that eight-year-old's fantasy. The breezes were warm and wet at the same time. The ocean waves looked inviting one minute and menacing the next, creating a dramatic visual I couldn't take my eyes away from. The sand was soft and fine, and I loved how the tiniest bits stuck all along the back of my legs when I laid on the beach. I paddleboarded in the bay and even had a spontaneous sighting of Anthony Kiedis of the Red Hot Chili Peppers. I truly felt like I was in paradise.

A tiny bit of that paradise did end up coming home with me: I gave birth to my first child, a beautiful girl, nine months later. And while everything about her has been perfect, the journey with her father was difficult. Pele's curse, said to bring bad luck to anyone who sneaks away with a physical piece of the island, like lava rocks or sand, seemed to have struck me. The first nine months of

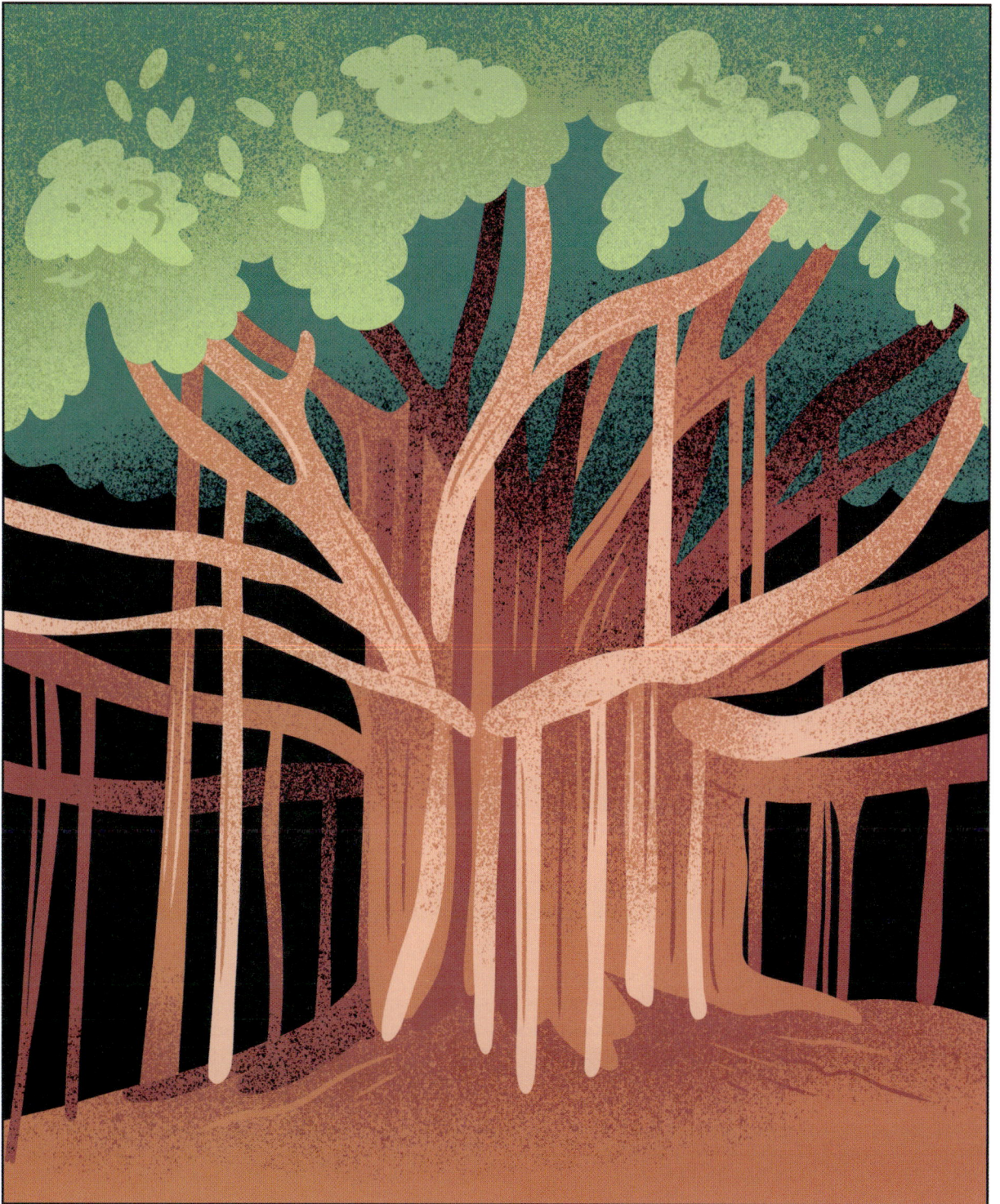

my daughter's life had been a juxtaposition between utter bliss as a new mom and complete emotional gutting as my relationship burned to the ground—surely the goddess's destructive fiery forces were to blame. The following year, I was exhausted and all I could think about was the soft embrace of Hawaii's wind, waves, and sand.

I have a photo of my nine-month-old daughter at the base of Lahaina's banyan tree. She is wearing a white onesie with ruffled cap sleeves. She is tan, fat, bald, and happy, showing off her gummy smile. She is completely unaware of my broken heart and the waves of anxiety I was riding in my life. That day, in search of a refuge, we found ourselves underneath the banyan's umbrella of foliage. Under this mystical, ancient guardian of the town, I watched my daughter totter around and place her hands on the bark that had been smoothed by a thousand other hands. Whose hands? I wondered. I watched my daughter's eyes thoughtfully contemplate what she saw when she looked up, expecting sky, but only saw branches of green. I sat longer and remembered that Buddha had apparently reached enlightenment while sitting under a banyan tree. I wondered if Buddha and Pele were friends. I did notice that I was breathing in a slow and steady way. And beginning to feel hope.

As a lover of all things plant and medicine, Ayurvedic practices streamed into my consciousness early on in my career. The traditional ways of using plant medicine, meaning approaches older than two hundred years, are particularly interesting to me. This is mainly because they emphasize the need to understand why something is happening in the body as much as what to use to treat it.

Digging into someone's symptoms in this way creates a story and timeline for pathology. It also provides keen insight to the patient, their bodily functions and level of organ function.

I'll use my own children as an example. I have two kids. My daughter is tall, slim, processes quickly, and is always cold. My son, on the other hand, is also slim but runs hot and his body processes slowly (in terms of digestion, detoxification). When the latest head-cold germ breaches our house, even if it is the same virus, they will present symptoms very differently. My daughter will have a perpetual runny nose, thin mucous with very little color. My son will always end up completely congested with thick, yellow mucous. Knowing their bodies' differences in function allows me to treat them more efficiently—I won't give them the same remedies. I curate their treatment to alleviate their specific symptoms relative to body constitution.

This is the beauty of most traditional medicine philosophies such as Ayurvedic and Oriental medicine. In Ayurveda, there are three main types of body constitutions: vatta, pitta, and kapha. Vatta is associated with a fast metabolism and quick mind. They are on-the-go people, creative and energetic. Pitta types have a high metabolism, medium build, and internally run warm. They are ambitious and have a strong will but can be prone to inflammation. Kapha types are typically larger in size but not necessarily obese. They just have a heavier build and slower metabolism. They are often calm and loving but have a tendency toward lethargy. The banyan tree specifically has been used for medicine in Ayurvedic tradition because it offers something for all three body types. Several species of ficus, however, are used in traditional herbalism. Depending on where you are in the world, accounts for medicinal species are readily available.

This large evergreen with a fluted trunk is proficient at fruit and seed production. The seeds are dispersed by various animals and birds. Once germinated, wherever they land, seedlings begin as epiphytes that eventually put down roots that often kill the original host, hence its common name of "strangler fig." It is monoecious and fast growing.

I find banyan leaves to be particularly beautiful. They are glossy green and 0.8 to 2.4 inches long. Their shape is ovate to elliptic with both the primary and lateral veins showing prominently. They also have fuzzy petioles that are fun to touch. Flowers arrive in spring, but Ficus benghalensis doesn't bloom like a normal flowering tree—I learned from the Tula House in Brooklyn, New York, that ficus flowers are actually inside the fruit! This makes them very unique, and shows how clever their coevolutionary relationship is with their main pollinators: wasps.

So many of us are taught to hate and kill wasps, but there are so many valuable wasp pollinators. It is vitally important to recognize that they support our fragile plant world. The specialized female *Eupristina masoni* wasp pollinates banyans by squeezing her way into the ostiole at the bottom of the fig, often losing both her wings and her antennae in the process. Once inside, she pollinates the internal stigmas and lays her eggs among the hundreds of internal inflorescences. Her job complete, she dies. As a result, the flowers bear seeds and a new generation begins.

Banyan Recipes

INDICATIONS

- Arthritis
- Asthma
- Bronchitis
- Burn healing
- Coughs
- Diabetes
- Diarrhea
- Gastric ulcers
- Gum bleeding
- Managing infection
- Nausea
- Protection from oxidative damage
- Wound healing

*Generally regarded as safe for all populations, but not to be used fresh. Stomach discomfort with excess intake has been reported; ensure fruits are dried before consumption due to the laxative effect of fresh fruit.

MORNING LATTE

Research has shown that if we drink insulin-supporting herbs first thing in the morning, before eating, they support balanced blood sugar and reduce sugar cravings all day long. Whether you are working to reduce sugar intake in your daily diet or you tend to have big swings in your glucose throughout the day, this latte may help.

Items needed:
Saucepan
Stirring spoon
2-cup measuring cup
8-cup measuring cup
Electric drink mixer
Frother (optional)
Tea mug

Ingredients:
10 oz. water
3.5 oz of milk (any type)
½ tsp. of banyan tree bark powder
½ tsp. of dandelion root powder
¼ tsp. ground cinnamon
¼ tsp. ground ginger
¼ tsp. ground cardamom
½ tsp. vanilla extract
1 tsp. maple syrup or honey

Put all dried ingredients into the large glass measuring cup and pour the boiling water over it.

Use the electric drink mixer to blend and dissolve the powder in the water.

Add the vanilla and sweetener of your choice and mix again.

Pour into a tea mug.

Steam or froth the milk and add to the mug.

TOPICAL WART TREATMENT

Have you ever tried milking a tree before? The milk from the banyan tree has a long history of eliminating warts. Taking a small knife, such as a paring knife, make 2-to-3 inch cuts along the trunk or a branch. You'll immediately see milk seeping from the cut. Scoop the milk into a glass vial to collect it. (The leaves also contain milk, but I find it more difficult to collect this way. If you have easy access to a banyan tree, try plucking a leaf and tearing it in half; this will reveal the milk, which you can apply directly to the skin.)

Items needed:
Small, sharp knife
1-dram amber glass vial
Cotton swab

Once you've collected the banyan bark milk, use a cotton swab to apply it directly to the wart.

Apply three times a day for three weeks and then evaluate the wart's size and presence. Continue repeating treatment if needed, until the wart is removed.

Beech

Fagus americana,
Fagus sylvatica,
Fagus grandifolia,
Fagus ferruginea

Family: Fagaceae
Parts used: flowers,
bark, and leaves
Medicinal actions:
antiseptic,
astringent, tonic
Native geography:
Fagus sylvatica:
Europe, particularly
Germany and England
Fagus grandifolia:
northern to eastern
America; now wide-
spread across the US

Some trees are just burned into your memory forever, even if they don't feature in a specific story or important event; sometimes their consistent presence in the background just makes them an essential part of the arc of your life. A beech grew in the gravel Dairy Queen parking lot by my home, and I remarked it because it grew straight up, right out of a 4-by-4-foot patch of grass only protected from dogs by a low, two-beam wood fence. The parking lot was regularly refreshed with white gravel rock that created a perpetual plume of dust. As a kid I didn't think much about this tree besides how feeling the gritty dust on the leaves gave me an icky feeling. But it did offer shade during the hottest (and most humid) days of Nebraska summers as we desperately tried to eat our ice creams before they melted.

As a kid, I was afforded the luxury of waking up slowly and naturally every day of summer break. There is very little that compares to the peace and joy of this simple act. No alarm, no person or parent rousing you. Just those precious moments when you realize, gradually, that you are waking up. Maybe you hear a bird sing, or distant noises from the kitchen. But without urgency, you can stretch or pull your knees up to your chest and wrap the blankets over you for just a bit longer. After I fully opened my eyes I'd lazily contemplate whether I was ready to begin a new day or roll over and go back to sleep. I cherished summer vacation. My mom had gone back to work when I was nine and I didn't assume any real responsibility until I was thirteen, which meant I had four glorious years of embracing

all the freedom that being a kid in summer had to offer.

It was the 1980s, and mom fed us Cheerios, Wheaties, and Chex during the school year, but in the summer she replaced those with Lucky Charms, Frosted Flakes, or Cap'n Crunch. Most days it was already eighty-plus degrees by the time I woke up, so I'd make my way to the back of the house where our TV was, in a room where the sun's burning rays hadn't yet reached. I would scoot our 1970s captain's chair close enough to the screen that I could rest my feet on the TV stand and prop my cereal on my knees, so I could turn the channel if I needed to without getting up.

I'd start most mornings watching *The Price Is Right*, fascinated by memorizing the prices of grocery store items despite never having to buy so much as a tube of toothpaste. I even had a fantasy of bidding one dollar when everyone else had overbid, and I'd jump and scream my way on stage. Next came *The Young and the Restless*, and by the time it aired my sister would have made her way downstairs, munching her own bowl of cereal and give me side-eye, daring me to try and change the channel. So I'd mosey around at this point until I got bored enough to endure the rising summer swelter waiting for me outside. I can still feel the way the heat hit me the moment I'd open the back door—it instantly penetrated every cell in my body and brain. Though I would also be temporarily blinded from the brightness of the sun and my lungs would heave in the humidity, I hit the pavement to see what was buzzing in the neighborhood. Which unfortunately, was never very

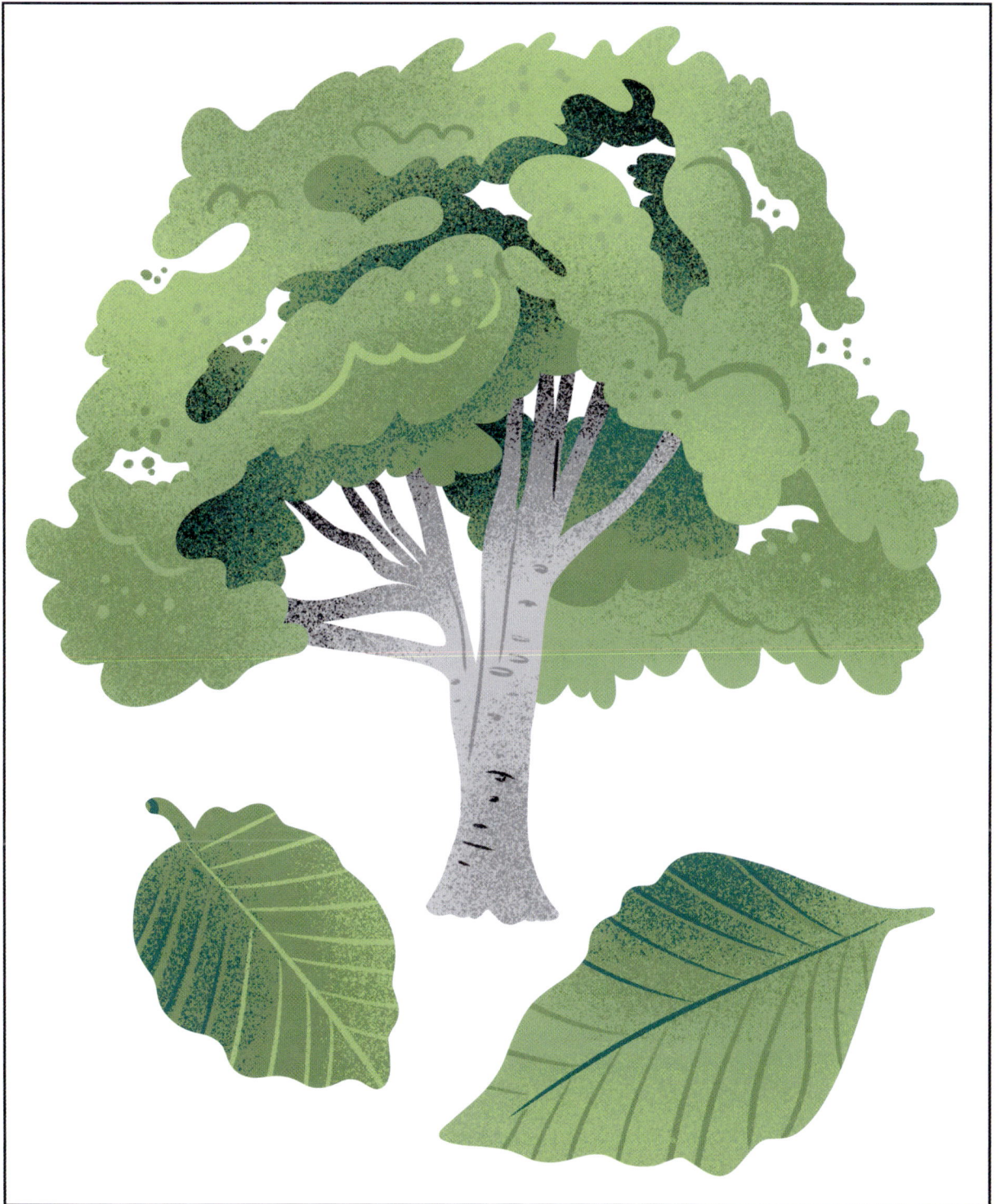

**USDA hardiness
zones:** 3 to 9
Water: keep
moderately damp
Light requirement:
shade to partial shade
Soil: prefers moist, rich,
and well-drained soil but
can grow in sandy, clay
and loam-rich soils
Temperature: frost
tolerant to -20° F
Wildlife notes: nuts are
a favorite food for squirrels, raccoons, bears,
and game birds
Pollinator friendly: bees,
butterflies, and moths all
use spring beech pollen
as an early food source
Pests: wooly beech
aphids, oyster beech
scale, beetles

much. Most of my neighbors were geriatric homeowners who were friendly enough but not playmates.

I'd save the change I found—fair game if someone just left it out on the coffee table, by my logic—carefully adding it to my little velcro coin purse. And once I had $1.25, there was no doubt where I was headed: Dairy Queen. The building was a square of large cement blocks, plopped in the middle of that gravel lot, painted white with a red roof and had the old-school walk-up window that the employees would slide open only when they had to, to keep the cool air in. Most kids would come tearing in there on their bikes, skidding to a halt before throw-ing their bikes on the ground. I always dis-mounted before I hit the gravel because I was scared of how the gravel grabbed my tires.

The beech was around the back. To me, it always seemed a bit out of place, alone in a parking lot. I wondered if it had just sprouted there or if someone had intentionally planted it. Beech trees are funny because they are often tall but dome-shaped, so from far away they give the appearance of having a short trunk. Sitting on the one coveted bench underneath it, you could lean back with your ice cream cone and see that the trunk actually stretched all the way up to the sky. On those special summer days, we would meet up under that beech tree to catch a moment of shade and plan the day's adventure.

A favorite of lovers, beech seems to be one of the most-graffitied trees of our time. There is something attractive about the smooth gray wood and how, once the names are carved in it, the bark reveals the engraver's initials clearly, conveying bold intent. Unlike other trees, the beech's bark rarely changes color or

texture as it ages, so the names endure.

The beech is a sturdy and imposing tree with an easily identifiable trunk. They often remind me of an elephant's foot, with their bumpy toes and one mighty leg. It is also identified by its often perfectly rounded crown of horizontal outstretched branches and dense growth.

The leaves are 6 to 12cm long, dark green and glossy on top and lighter green under-neath. They are deeply veined and in the fall the leaves turn a bright copper to light up the short days. Every two or three years, the tree also produces beechnuts in the fall. They look a bit like lychee fruit and are best described as a prickly bur containing triangular brown and shiny nuts. These nuts are crucial in many wildlife winter food stores.

Beech has a long and interesting history when it comes to medicinal use. A favorite of the Iroquois tribe, it was often employed to cleanse the blood, heal skin afflictions, and was used for respiratory conditions that were classified as "wet" in nature, such as pneumonia. It's listed among the pages of *Culpeper's Complete Herbal* and John King's work for similar conditions, with the addition of wood tar, or creosote—it now seems archaic to consider inhaling or ingesting tar, but it was a popular respiratory and sinus remedy in the nineteenth century.

Beech still shines in the mental/emo-tional areas of medicine. In herbal medicine, we call "flower essences" medicines that treat imbalances on the energetic level. While my practice is rooted in scientific medi-cine, occasionally I find value and truth in what the "woo-woo" practitioners promote. The Flower Essence Society (FES) has been researching plant energetics since the early 1970s, continuing Dr. Edward Bach's work of the 1930s. Anyone who studies the body and medicine knows, at some point the question arises "Which came first, the physical pathology or an emotional imbalance?" When I meet with patients, we often dive into their life history, including an evaluation of what areas of their lives are happy and what areas are not. The unhappy areas are scored to help identify how much stress those unhappy parts add. That stress might manifest as anxiety, anger, depression, etc. What clinical research has proven is that repeated stress, in whatever form or from whatever vector, does have the ability to change how our body functions. It can change our cells, even turn genes on or off.

Our mental and emotional well-being is just as important as physical health, and I believe that our physical health is much stronger when we are happy. The FES believes this also. Through research, they have identified plants that affect our mental/emotional selves. Beech, one of the original thirty-eight flower essences researched by Dr. Bach, has an affinity for those who tend to be hypercritical of themselves and others. Perhaps you have a past where you were never allowed to freely be who you wanted to be. Maybe you experienced a lot of judgment from others or were never praised for your positive attributes. As a result, you could have learned critical behaviors and carried them forth into your adult life. This often leads to intolerance of others with little compassion for understanding or appreciating others' differences. Beech flower essence can help.

Often we blend flower essences together to address a particular issue someone is struggling with, frequently a child's nightmares, overt physical trauma, or self-deprecation. You might be familiar with the most popular flower essence, sold under the commercial name Rescue Remedy. It's a household staple for me, and we take it for any traumatic event, no matter how big or small. If taken during acute stress it can instantly calm and slow down revved-up reactions to stressful situations. It's great for pets, too.

Beech Recipes

————

INDICATIONS

- Burns
- Chronic eczema
- Critical feelings or moods
- Diarrhea
- Dysentery
- Frostbite
- Indigestion
- Low-grade fevers
- Respiratory illness

*Tar is no longer considered safe in the United States, but it is interesting to note that Eldon Boyd, a Canadian chemist, experimented in his lab with one of the active constituents in beech tar, guaiacol. Its derivate, glycerol guaiacolate, is more commonly known as guaifenesin, now one of the most common ingredients in over-the-counter cold medicines including Mucinex, Robitussin, and DayQuil.

Historically the nut has been a food source, but be sure to research before consumption as nausea and vomiting have occurred after eating.

BEECH LEAF CORDIAL

This cordial recipe is technically a beech leaf noyau, an alcohol-based drink (or apple cider vinegar–based, when it can be used as an aperitif or digestif). A cordial is a medicinal tonic that stimulates the organs to improve circulation. When you activate the organs of the body in this way, you help to move out the sludge or toxins that may have accumulated. They are low in sugar and also have a positive impact on your digestive system. This is in part due to the healthy bacteria and enzymes that are a result of the fermentation process. In Shakespeare's day, a cordial was referred to as any medicine used to stimulate the heart, but of course a poet would say that!

The word noyau comes from French, meaning the stones of fruits, or stone fruits: plums, apricots, peaches. Beech noyau is said to have originated with the forest workers of the Chiltern hills of England during the eighteenth century, but I'm not exactly sure how the name stuck with the substitution of beech leaves versus stone fruits. Either way, drink responsibly, either neat or over ice.

Items needed:
One-liter glass jar with lid
Storage bottles of your choice, glass preferred

Ingredients:
Fresh, young beech leaves
32-oz. bottle of gin, brandy, or apple cider vinegar
    (or combine two of these fluids)
8.5 oz. distilled water
8.8 oz. organic cane sugar

Pack the jar with the freshly collected beech leaves. They should be newly sprouted and bright green in color. Fill the jar with your liquid of choice and close tightly.

Shake vigorously for one minute.

Store in a cool, dark place for three weeks, shaking the jar every few days.

Strain and pour into smaller storage bottles. Be sure to label your bottles with contents and date.

BEECH LEAF CHIPS

Move over kale chips, there's a new crisp in town. Here is another unique way to use beech leaves that creates a medicinal snack.

Items needed:
Large mixing bowl
Stirring spoon
Cookie tray
Airtight storage container

Ingredients:
3 cups fresh beech leaves
3 tbsp. olive oil
2 tbsp. nutritional yeast
Sprinkle of salt and pepper

Preheat the oven to 250 to 270° F. Put all ingredients in the mixing bowl and stir well. Lay leaves out in a single layer on the cooking tray and bake for 20 to 25 minutes, until they are crispy but not charred. Allow to cool before eating. If there are any leftovers, store them in an airtight container.

Bonsai

Ulmus parvifolia, Ficus retusa, Juniperus sp. and *Acer palmatum* are commonly trained as bonsai, but almost any tree or shrub can be used

Medicinal actions:
Nervine

The farmer gently bent over a small ceramic pot. I watched as his eyes pored over the miniature tree, scrutinizing, evaluating, and determining which leaves to trim and where to place his pruning shears. His head moved slowly, side to side, looking at it from every angle. There was a precision in his movements and actions that spoke to years of muscle memory at this task.

One day I made us tea. It was afternoon, early summer. The sun dipped behind the clouds from time to time, and because temperatures were still climbing, a cup of tea to recharge had felt like the right thing to do. He loved an herbal blend called Evening in Missoula, one of those teas with a flavor so unique that every time you drink it, it recalls the memory of the first time you had it. A combination of citrus, mints, fruits, and flowers that slowed the body and stimulated the mind.

I had arrived on the farm as a volunteer. I was hoping my zeal for manual labor would outweigh my general lack of experience with large-scale herb farming. I had always been a hard worker. I am on the shorter side, five foot three, but built solid like an ox. Someone once told me that our thighs are indicative of our occupation in a previous life; she followed this statement up by saying I must have been a farmer.

Working outside has always felt satisfying to me: digging, raking, planting, watering, lifting, cleaning. I like the way my body feels afterward, and the sense of accomplishment. I like the honest exchange: I contribute energy, and in and in return the land gives me something back. I like immersing myself in the elements, keeping my mind connected to the seasons and maintaining my body to adapt to change. But most of all, it is the connection I feel with the environment. It really doesn't matter how many times I see a seedling pop free from the soil—it never gets old. The same goes for turning over an old log or bark piece and marveling at all the life teeming underneath. Even now, in my fifties, I am still in awe of all that the natural world has created around us.

On that farm, at first I just did everything as I was told. In the barn, an ancient but well-maintained, gambrel-roofed building, a to-do list was written on a whiteboard. For me, one of the best things about most farm jobs is that you can jump in without a lot of fuss or explanation. Most chores are straightforward: choose one and get to work. Granted, most of the things on this whiteboard were for those of us new to the team, which meant the tasks chosen were ones the farmer felt fairly confident we couldn't mess up.

He was a tall man, the owner of the farm. He didn't talk too much, but had an ease about him that made others open up in his presence. He welcomed us all up to the porch at the end of the day for a cold drink and a bit of chin-wagging. He'd smile and give us glimmers of his life—we could never quite piece it together. At some point we'd all drift away and leave him there, with the sun setting over his left shoulder.

After a few months, I had apparently proven myself. He asked me to join his hired team in preparation for the season. He also

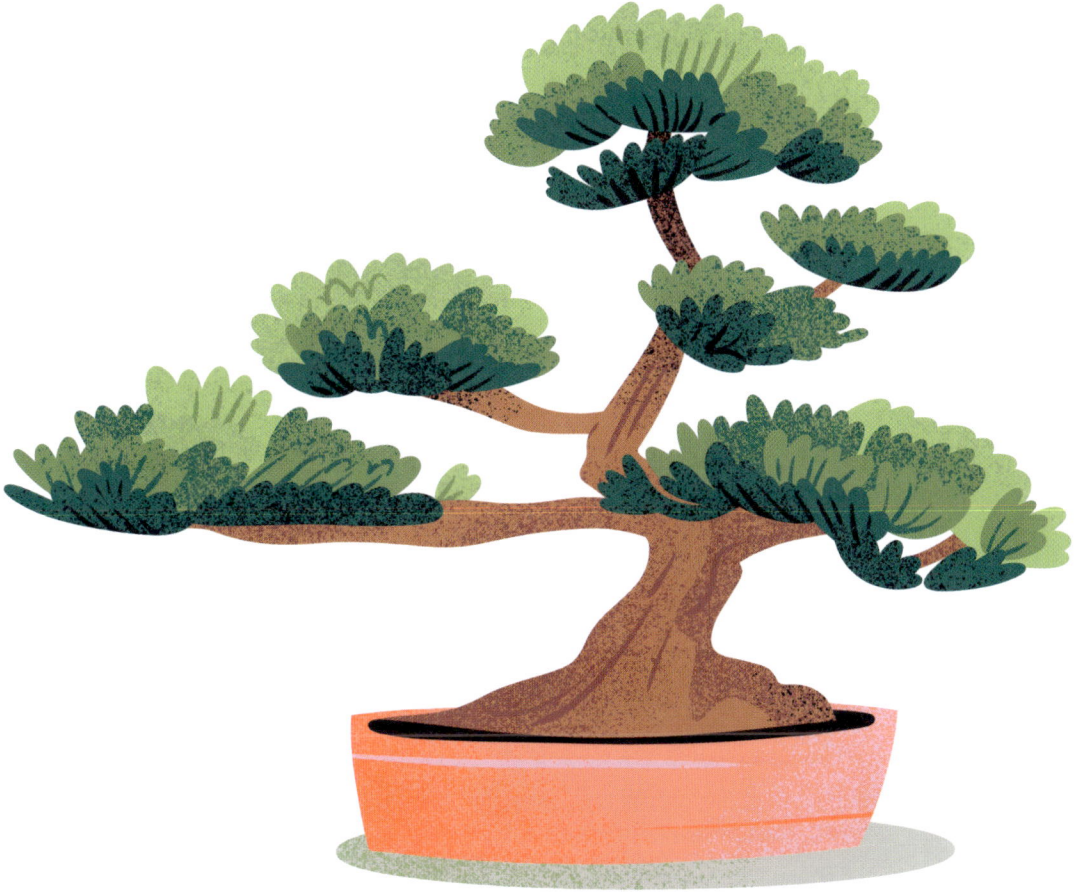

USDA hardiness zones: typically grown indoors; can be grown outdoors in a zones 7 to 9

Water: water before soil gets dry but don't over-water; do not water on a strict routine, but check moisture by inserting your finger into the soil about half an inch deep. If it feels dry, water

Light requirement: part shade, shade

Soil: the soil mixture greatly influences how often trees need to be watered; most bonsai trees thrive on a mixture of akadama, pumice, and lava rock in a ratio of two parts to one part to one part; calcium carbonate (limestone) tolerance is low

Temperature: tropical tree species need relatively high temperatures throughout the year, around 60 to 75° F and they prefer humidity; mist your bonsai daily to support the latter

Pollinator friendly: pollinators particularly love the dwarf powder puff

Pests: aphids, mealy bugs, spider mites, vine weevils

asked whether I could house-sit for a few days while he went to visit his sister. He knew I loved the quiet of the land—as well as the dog that followed me around most days. He said he needed someone there "in case something happened." I asked what could possibly go wrong. "Oh, a water main might break, or a spontaneous fire could break out. . ." he said calmly and with a blank face. I mustered non-chalance in return but I frantically wondered how in the hell I'd handle something like that. "And one other thing," he said. "I need you to keep an eye on my bonsai."

I thought back to how I had seen him delicately caring for that plant, his giant hands holding tiny shears and giving a precise snip from time to time. Someone had said it was a family heirloom, that it had been passed down for generations and now resided with him. I thought of the two times I had tried bonsai gardening, both ending in plant death because I had pretended to know how to care for them instead of actually taking time to learn the intricate care they require. I immediately worried that I could bring his beloved bonsai to its demise in just a few days, but I pushed those thoughts out of my mind.

Later, I stood before the bonsai and begged it to be patient with me. I acknowledged I was not emitting the energy it was used to, but if it could at the very least stay in stasis, alive, I would be eternally grateful. I didn't dare use the shears, but I gently raked around its trunk to show I cared. Together, we survived.

———————

In my last years of graduate school I focused on chronic diseases, oncology, and hospice care. While my treatments included acupuncture and education around supportive care, most of my time was spent simply sitting and listening to patients. When we are faced with extreme health challenges and/or our own mortality, there is an honesty that usually overcomes us. As a result many of these patients talked freely about their lives—some of them for the first time ever.

Regret is defined as feeling sad, repentant, or disappointed over something that has happened or been done, especially a loss or missed opportunity. I think to some degree we all have regrets. Conversations we wish had gone differently, choices we wish we would or would not have made. And while we mostly chalk these up to naiveté, youth, or ignorance, the problem is that some regrets can be very difficult to let go. Regrets cause suffering. When we hold on to an event that challenged us, brought us anger, grief, or unexpected devastation, it finds a way to live inside of us. Say what you will, but as a trained and experienced health care practitioner, I've seen patients' internal suffering manifest as illness. We all know that stress can cause stomach ulcers and drives up blood pressure, for example. Strong feelings preoccupy our brain and affect parts of our physical makeup. Learning to process and release them is one aspect of regaining peace and balance in health. In Western society, we are often taught to suppress our emotions and not to challenge others, even in a nonconfrontational manner. As children we are told to buck up, hold our chins up, that doing hard things makes us stronger. Rarely is space created where we simply say, "That really sucked. Want a hug?" As a result, we tuck our pain away.

While this book definitely focuses on the medicinal qualities of trees, bonsai isn't used internally as medicine. The reason I included it is due to the practice's association with mental health benefits. There is something uniquely special about cultivating a bonsai tree. The relationship that is formed is one of giving and receiving, the type of relationship that everyone benefits from. The bonsai gives joy, fascination, and a sense of satisfaction while you create a suitable environment and cultivate the practice of tending to its needs. Because there is such closeness, you'll notice every time a new branch sprouts or leaves bud out. It is a mutual recognition of accomplishment and gratitude.

The need to find outlets to release damaging inner dialogues is crucial. There are many ways to help us do this: exercise, meditation, therapy, and bodywork such as Rosen therapy just to name a few. I've included bonsai here as another option. To connect with another living thing in the delicate and enduring practice of bonsai, can really help. The act of tending to a bonsai tree can foster calmness and serenity. It requires detailed care, enhances concentration, and allows you to escape to the solace of the present moment. Even five minutes of this activity can change brain chemistry. I suggest using it as a therapist.

While caring for your bonsai, notice what it needs and also share what is at the forefront of your mind: talk to it. Verbalizing thoughts gets them out of the loop inside your head. Physically moving with care and precision while releasing thoughts and feelings can shift them out of your body. And while the other previously mentioned release techniques are great, getting a bonsai is a low-barrier way to begin the emotional release process.

So what did most of my chronic disease and hospice patients talk about while I sat with them? Typically, yes, it did often start with regrets. But as old stories that occupied too many cobwebbed corners in their brain began getting swept away, their moods improved and so did their physical symptoms. They freely shared the pain of their lives, but could now do it with humor and wisdom. They released all their regrets because they now knew there was no place for them anymore. We all have regrets, but as they had discovered, regrets are not to be held on to, reserved to perpetuate an endless cycle of suffering. They are simply experiences. Looking at them can help us to better understand ourselves and forgive ourselves so that we can move on, in peace.

Bonsai Recipes

INDICATIONS

- Anxiety
- Depression
- Grief
- Stress

Interestingly enough, while the word "bonsai" originates from Japanese, the practice and art of creating bonsai is an ancient Chinese agricultural practice. Translated, it means "planted in a shallow container." There are three main types of traditional bonsai trees: broadleaf evergreen, deciduous, and coniferous. The ficus is considered the easiest species to care for and is a good choice for a budding bonsai enthusiast.

BONSAI SOIL

Bonsai trees require regular watering and fertilizing. Fertilization is important since it lives in a container. Bonsais need adequate nitrogen, phosphorus, potassium, iron, magnesium, and zinc. We often only think about nitrogen for strong leaf and shoot growth, but trace minerals such as potassium help with photosynthesis. Since the bonsai root system is so much smaller than a regular tree, it is easy to overwhelm and damage it with overfertilization. Using a slow-release fertilizer is the way to go.

FERTILIZER BALLS

Best to be made outdoors, due to smell.

Items needed:
Mixing bowl
Disposable gloves
Wax paper
Small airtight storage container

Ingredients:
4 cups cottonseed meal
2 cups bonemeal
1 cup fish meal
⅓ cup kelp meal
2 cups fish emulsion
½ cup liquid fertilizer, adjust depending on moisture needs

Mix everything together with your hands in the mixing bowl. Adjust liquid fertilizer amounts until you achieve a consistency like cookie dough. Roll portions into 1-inch balls, then flatten. Lay them out on wax paper to dry and then store in an airtight container.

As soon as the growing season begins in spring, add a fertilizer ball to the soil. It will slowly break down each time you water.

MUCK ADHERENT

Muck is used as a type of "glue" to secure slabs and stone around and/
or with a bonsai. It holds everything in place like a self-adhering clay
that then hardens after it dries. A good recipe creates a strong muck
that is also permeable so water and roots can penetrate as needed. It
can also be used to create an edging to retain the bonsai soil in the pot.

Items needed:
Mixing bowl
Mixing spoon
Disposable gloves

Ingredients:
1 cup bentonite
5 cups high-grade compost manure
1 cup sphagnum moss
Water

Add the bentonite, compost, and sphagnum all together. Using your
hands, mash and mix well. If needed, cut the sphagnum moss into small
pieces to make it easier to mix. Slowly add ½ cup of water at a time and
mix well. The compound should feel slightly sticky, yet easy to handle. It
should also hold itself up and retain a shape.

Cedar

Thuja occidentalis,
Thuja plicata

Family: Cupressaceae
Parts used: leaves,
essential oil
Medicinal actions:
antibacterial, antifungal,
anti-inflammatory,
antioxidant, antiviral,
emmenagogue,
expectorant
Native geography:
eastern and central
Canada and the eastern
and north-central
portions of the
United States

*"To sit in solitude, to
think in solitude with
only the music of the
stream and the cedar
to break the flow of
silence, there lies the
value of wilderness."*
—John Muir

When out in my beloved nearby woods, I'll often see a white-tailed deer near a white northern cedar; it's a favorite. My friend Don, a member of the Apache Nation, once told me their story of how deer get their spots. As the legend goes, a new mother will position her fawns next to a burning fire made of cedar. Anywhere a cracking or popping ember lands on its fur will create a spot. When he told me this story, I was myself almost nine months pregnant with my daughter. I had recently been thinking a lot about the impending labor process as I'd reached that point in pregnancy where it could be "go time" at any moment. My brain often fluctuated between terror and the complete fantasy that I would breeze through the process.

Close to where I was living then, there was a park with a nice footpath. I would walk from my house through old neighborhoods on cracked sidewalks no one had the time to repair. I'd look at the same porches, gardens, and yard art almost every single day. First would be the house with the ever-revolving door of new tenants with a front porch almost as saggy as the couch sitting on it. There was the garden of wild native plants; the owner was one of the first in our area to have ripped up the grass in an attempt to make the yard more environmentally friendly. There were the two pit bulls inside a chain-link fence on the corner. When they heard my footsteps from down the street they'd bark but then instantly stop and wait, with their fat long tongues hanging out, for their daily pets. I would see the same people coming and going from their homes, or notice them inside their houses doing the same sorts of tasks I do at home. It felt like I knew them, but I didn't really know them at all.

It made me think about the little person inside of me and how I didn't know her at all either. Despite cohabitating for almost nine months, I didn't know what foods she would like, her eye color, or whether she enjoyed the music I often played for her. My biggest question was something much deeper and attached to my biggest fear: What if we didn't like each other? What if I couldn't handle being a mom and instead of acting compassionately toward her, I started to feel resentment? What if she was just disagreeable and unpleasant to be around? When you are nine months pregnant with your first child, so many crazy thoughts come up.

Thankfully I used the park as a place I knew I could visit to remind me to breathe deeply and relax, which would in turn help return my mind to a more rational state. On days when my thoughts started to spiral, I'd ignore the pain in my hips and waddle my way to Fernhill Park. There, I'd find my favorite bench among the cedar trees and look out over rolling hills. There is something majestic and graceful about the structure of a cedar tree. Their slender spray of branches reached out all around and above me which felt like the safety of a mother's embrace. I'd stare upwards through boughs, projecting my thoughts as if they were listening and ready to offer advice and wisdom. I'd clip tiny bits from their tips to chew and suck on as I'd contemplate this wild new adventure I was on. The cedars helped me muster up enough clarity to plow onward.

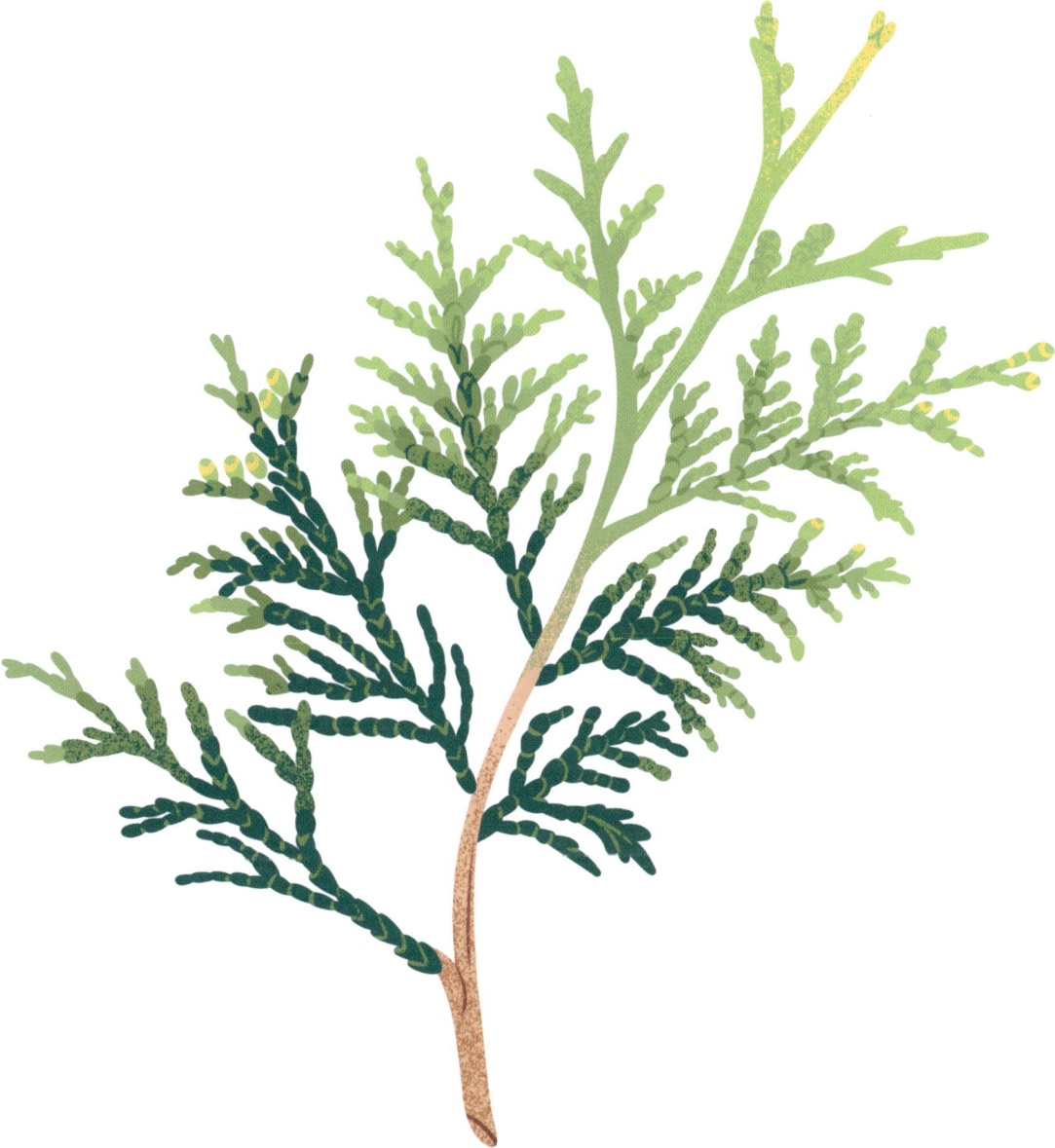

PLANT DATA

USDA hardiness zones: 2 to 9

Water: water as needed as a seedling, but avoid overwatering at young ages as this subjects it to fungal infections; once established it's relatively drought tolerant

Light requirement: full sun to shade

Soil: neutral or slightly alkaline soils derived from limestone, but it can grow in clay, loamy and sandy soil

Temperature: cold hardy

Wildlife notes: white-tailed deer use it for food and shelter

Pollinator friendly: wind-pollinated

Pests: few; the resin in northern white cedar (NWC) protects against insects, mold, and mildew

Maybe it's regular first-pregnancy jitters, maybe it's hormones or fear of the unknown, but thankfully all of those uncertainties flew out the window the moment I met my daughter. And then again, later with my son. The one thing that did carry over from that time period is my connection to cedar. When I started conceiving this book, cedar was the first tree I thought to include; but it was actually the last entry I wrote, which seems appropriate. Cedar trees hold a key place in my soul that brings on a feeling of peace and connection to myself. Is this a remnant of a collective memory? Did my forebears believe that the spirits of our ancestors live in the cedars, and that is why they bring such comfort to me? The answers will surely be revealed when my time comes, but until then I can only hypothesize why cedar has been firmly rooted in many key moments in my life.

My son walks the woods with me now and is quick to offer a cedar tip to suck on as we walk down the trail. My daughter hugs cedars like they're old friends when we come across them on our journeys. In my own way, like the white-tailed deer, I've done my best to initiate them into all the benefits that cedars offer. This way, when I'm gone, they can go to the cedar and feel my mother's embrace.

There is nothing I like more than to clip off a pinch of cedar to chew on while I'm walking in the woods. The flavor is much as you'd expect, aromatic and pungent on the tongue. It provides a cleansing, crisp feel in the mouth. It's lovely to have something we can all now silently share as we wander through the woods.

Once used with care internally, most herbalists these days will not recommend it. Cedar is high in volatile oils and one in particular,

thujone, can be toxic. In general volatile oils are not toxic—you may have used rosemary and lavender yourself. When a plant has a high volatile oil content, it is usually distilled to create essential oil. This process separates the oil from the water in the plant. Because ingestion of excess thujone blocks gamma aminobutyric acid (GABA), it can cause restlessness, excitability, insomnia, and tremors. The human body also struggles with processing thujone and it can damage the liver and kidneys when taken in excess. As with many historic medicines, healers struggled with the fine line of a dosage that would help or hurt. Many plants were taken to clean or purge the body; cedar, lobelia, and castor are a few commonly used. But because there is little education concerning how and when to use such medicinals, it is best to consult a professional before use. Be sure to check out the National Library of Medicine for research on internal uses.

This conifer is a slow and steady grower with shallow roots that tend to spread. A great choice for edging property and wildlife landscapes, they have sweeping branches that present green, scaled-looking, flat, fanlike foliage. It grows in a pyramidal shape and its foliage is dense, which makes for a great wind block in winter. It seems to command its space; you'll rarely see other plants or even weeds growing directly underneath it. If you happen to be near Lake Superior in Minnesota, be sure to stop by the Witch Tree, a cedar growing out of a cliff face. Originally written about in 1731 by the French explorer Sieur de la Vérendrye, it is still alive today.

One of the oldest uses of cedar tincture is for the treatment of skin warts. Apply it topically, three times a day for three weeks. I recommend applying a bit of cream around the wart to protect the surrounding skin and then use a small paintbrush to target where you dab the tincture. Some prefer to use the essential oil for this treatment, but I have found the tincture to be more successful.

That being said, the essential oil of cedar is a valuable tool for your medicine cabinet. It is great to add to the household diffuser to keep the air clean of bacteria and viral elements, particularly whenever someone in the house has a cold or guests are coming over for dinner. Cedar is also in my rotation for cold inhalation. Drop one to two drops into the palm of your hand, rub your hands together, and then breathe in deep. Then rub your hands around your neck and over your chest. It acts like a shield and gives microdoses of infection-fighting moments throughout the day whenever you catch a whiff.

Cedar essential oil is great for skin, too, particularly for burns and all inflammatory conditions. It calms and works to heal the underlying tissue. Speaking scientifically, cedar essential oil can affect gene expression. It does this by turning inflammatory genes off and supporting the immune and tissue remodeling response.

Cedar Recipes

INDICATIONS

- Abortiant
- Atherosclerosis
- Bronchitis
- Burns
- Cancer
- Colds
- Coughs
- Diabetes
- Digestive tonic
- Fevers
- Household
  cleaning spray
- Liver tonic
- Ringworm
- Tumors
- Warts
- Wounds

*Thujone is toxic in
  excessive doses—for
  external use only. Avoid
  if pregnant or nursing.*

BATH BLEND FOR CONGESTION

With all of the assaults our immune systems have recently faced, a
head cold sometimes barely registers as more than an inconvenience.
But if not treated, they can lead to a deeper pathology, such as a sinus
infection. There is something about a hot, steamy bath that always feels
good when I have a cold. While I often have to convince myself when
I'm run-down that it's worth the effort to draw the bath, undress, and
get into the tub, I force myself knowing it'll be beneficial.

Items needed:
Mixing bowl
Mixing spoon
Storage jar
Muslin bags

Ingredients:
3 cups Epsom salt
1 cup coarse sea salt
½ cup baking soda
2 tablespoons apricot kernel oil
1 cup chopped fresh white cedar leaves

Mix all the ingredients together in a bowl and then transfer into the
storage jar.

To use: Add 1 cup of mixture to a clean muslin bag and hang it over the
faucet so the water runs through it as you are filling the bathtub.

CEDAR BODY BALM

This balm has a multitude of uses. Place a smidge under the nose to help open up nasal passageways. Rub onto a sore joint, such as the shoulder or knee, for temporary relief. Great to heal dry and/or cracked cuticles.

Items needed:
Blender or herb grinder
Small saucepan, preferably with pour lip on the side
Small glass baking dish
Strainer
Storage bottle for oil
Glass jar for balm storage

Ingredients:
1 cup fresh cedar tips
½ oz. vodka or grain alcohol
8–12 oz. apricot oil
1 oz. beeswax
30 drops frankincense essential oil

Start by making a cedar-infused oil. To draw out the oils from the cedar, I recommend using the alcohol intermediary method below.

Collect 1 cup of fresh cedar tips and put them in a blender. Be sure your blender has a grind/finely chop setting; sometimes when you are making smaller amounts, the bigger blender blades can't cut up herbs very finely. Preferably you can get it to an almost powder stage.

Add the vodka and blend until it reaches the consistency of damp soil. Let this sit in the blender for 24 hours.

The next day, add your apricot oil and pulse a few times to get everything well mixed. Start with 8 oz.; if that is not enough to cover the herbal mixture or it doesn't seem loose, add a little more.

Pour this all into the glass baking dish and bake it at 150° F for 2 hours.

Strain and put 4 oz. of oil in the saucepan on low heat. Add ¾ to 1 oz. of beeswax, depending on how soft or hard you'd like your balm to be. Stir continuously until beeswax is melted, then remove it from heat. Swirl a few times to release a bit of heat and then add the frankincense essential oil. Swirl a few more times and pour it into a storage jar. Leave the lid off until completely cooled.

CEDAR SYRUP

This is an easy syrup to make that you can add to your favorite cocktail, mocktail, or culinary invention.

Items needed:
32-oz. mason jar
Teakettle
Strainer
Saucepan
Storage jar

Ingredients:
1 cup cedar tips
1 cup boiling water
1 cup sugar

Set the kettle to boil on the stove. In the meantime, cut the cedar tips into small ½-inch pieces and put them into the mason jar. Pour the boiling water over the top of the cedar and let steep, covered, overnight.

The next day, strain the cedar out from the liquid and transfer the liquid into the saucepan. Set the heat to low and add the sugar, stirring occasionally, until it is completely dissolved. Once dissolved, turn the heat up slightly and simmer for one minute.

Remove from the heat and pour into a storage bottle. Keep in the refrigerator and use within 1 to 2 weeks.

Ceiba

Ceiba pentandra

Family: Malvaceae
Parts used: leaves, flowers, roots, gum
Medicinal actions:
Bark: diuretic, emetic, purgative, tonic. *Roots:* diuretic, aphrodisiac, antipyretic. *Leaves:* emollient. *Flowers:* laxative. *Gum:* astringent, tonic, laxative. *Seed:* oil is antifungal, antibacterial, anti-inflammatory
Native geography:
Mexico, Central America and the Caribbean; northern South America, and West Africa; now also commonly found in Florida and Hawaii

I was 52 years years old when I finally made it to the Ecuadorian jungle, a place I had envisioned for as long as I could remember. My parents had always instilled a natural curiosity of the world beyond our Nebraska backyard. This was fostered by watching *Mutual of Omaha's Wild Kingdom* every Sunday night and with the stacks of *National Geographic* that went back decades that none of us could ever throw away. My mom would often find me sprawled out in the living room, on our orange shag carpet, with a smattering of various issues around me. Some would be open to full-page photographs while I perused the story of another. It was my version of traveling as a child. Wondering about these places and pretending what it would be like to experience them. I would get lost for hours in those pages and determined early on that I was marked for a life of adventure. I began my list of places to travel at age 4. Africa was first, and Ecuador would be second.

As someone who believes your soul is connected to the place of your conception, I've always held an affinity for Africa. A longing, you might say. My parents were living in Nigeria when I was conceived and I grew up hearing endless stories of what it was like to live there. (My parents moved back to the States before I was born.) Those stories are like ghosts of my past: a life I had, but also didn't. The black mamba snake that wrapped itself around the handle of my dad's tennis racket. The cook, who was always drunk, would eventually become blind with rage and chase the gardener with a machete. The pretty morning glory vines on the cottage where my family lived—the same vines that housed reptiles of all sorts that would sneak into the house at night. These stories also included the Ceiba trees, a tree that at the bottom looks like rivers and streams flowing out from the trunk and was so tall you rarely could see the top. I would imagine what it would be like to climb these trees. To reach the top and see the entire world. These stories of wildness and adventure, a life I felt meant for and one so different from my own. Perhaps this was one reason I was pulled into the *National Geographics*, time after time, craving the experiences of all walks of life.

If you are familiar with *National Geographic*, you know they loved spotlighting Africa throughout the years. But it was in the pages of an old archived issue where I discovered the Amazonian jungle. The Amazon jungle, also known as the Amazon rainforest, is primarily located in South America. It spans across nine countries: Brazil, Peru, Bolivia, Ecuador, Colombia, Venezuela, French Guiana, Guyana, and Suriname. A wild and vast place with multiple cultures, wildlife, and diverse ecosystems. And, as I flipped the page, Ecuadorian Ceiba trees. My beloved tree from the stories I'd been told since I was born. It was a photo of explorers standing next to the trunk of a giant tree. They looked like tiny men as the 200 feet tall tree loomed above them. A trunk with a flared buttress that showed deep grooves resembling rolling valley's on a mountainside. Here was my mystical tree, an actual photo of it. (Remember, this was 1979, there was no quick way to find images of things you were curious about.) My whole

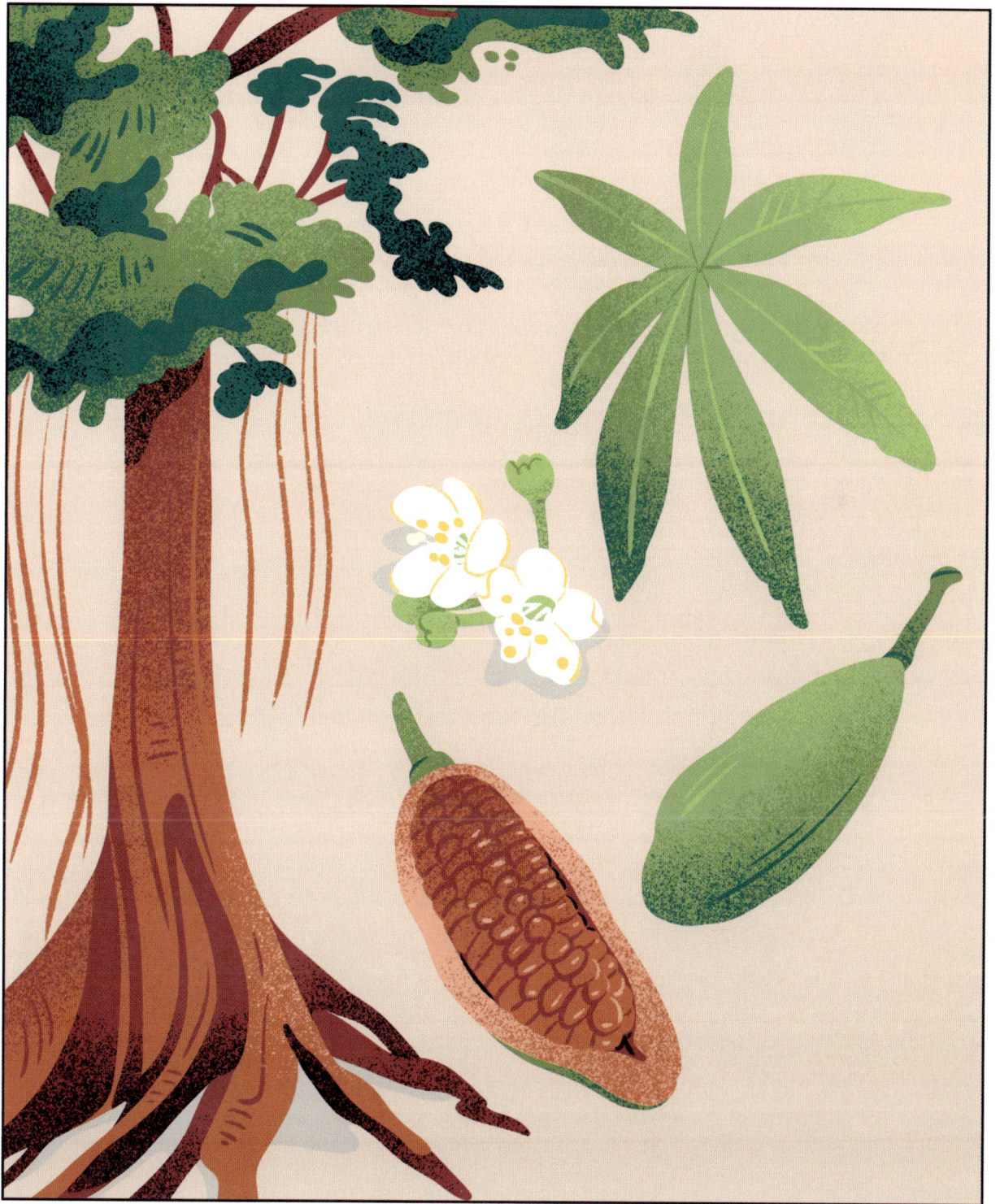

PLANT DATA
USDA hardiness
zones: 10 to 12
Water: abundant
moisture during their
vegetative period, less
moisture in winter or
during the dry season
Light requirement:
full sun
Soil: moist and
well-drained
Temperature:
intolerant of frost
Wildlife notes:
in a synergistic partner-
ship, bromeliads grow
on the ceiba, which
collect water and in
turn host frogs
Pollinator friendly:
pollinator bats visit
at night
Pests: termites
and fungi

body longed to feel the bark and to sit in one of those grooves for hours on end. My brain and heart exploded at this discovery and at age 7, I was ready to pack my bags for a visit. Maybe I'd bring a stack of *National Geographic* and camp out there all day, nestled against the trunk, sharing with it the stories and photo-graphs of the world.

Then, 45 years later, I made it. I took a flight, and then a smaller plane, to a bus and onto a boat. I stepped into a long peke peke boat on a wide and fast-flowing river and we headed downstream. Peke peke boats are low to the water, so I stuck my hand out to splash the coolness of the river as we moved along. I looked up and saw the endless jungle on either side of me and the giant ceiba trees standing taller than the rest. If only I could have been a bird for this one moment. I felt the trees watching me, as much as I was watch-ing them, calling me with joy at my arrival.

On this journey we visited the oldest ceiba tree of the region. A surprise on the itin-erary. As I approached and realized what I was about to witness, an incredible calm snaked its way into my soul. I breathed a breath deeper than my existence and opened up to the flow between all of creation. I slowly walked, in and out of the deep grooves of the trunk, lightly touching certain spots and embracing others. I stopped and pressed my entire being against it to feel its presence within. I slowed my heart and felt the pulse of ancient life. It was then that I realized, in another dimension, they, the ceiba's, had been silently witnessing my trans-formations as a person on this planet, perhaps guiding me more than I'll ever know.

———

Traditional herbal medicine comes from a long line of experienced herbalists, and from all cultures around the world. While

we do have a propensity to study and use the plants that grow in our own backyards, today we can take advantage of a worldwide pharmacy. When we learn about plants that grow in faraway regions, it also weaves the threads of the worldwide healing community together. Humans are complicated creatures, so it's taken centuries of trial and error to find remedies for what ails us. This is the one downfall of allopathic medicine. While it is a reasonable system to treat a mass population of people, having one approach in an attempt to heal doesn't necessarily take individuality into account.

For example, take David, a 63-year-old man who had been diagnosed with non-Hodgkin lymphoma. He showed up in my office for acupuncture and support treatment as he was undergoing chemotherapy and radiation. My focus was to keep side effects of the allopathic treatment down, as well as to support his energy levels and daily functioning. The one area where I couldn't gain traction, no matter what I tried, was his continued elevation in liver enzymes. He was the best patient and complied with every treatment plan suggested: tried and true botanicals, natural home treatments, exercise, and even, reluctantly, diet changes.

I was getting to my wits' end, like when you finish a puzzle but are missing the last piece. He was doing so great, but those pesky liver enzymes, I knew, would eventually cause more issues. So what do naturopaths do at this point? We don't give up. That is, in my opinion, one of the best things about a good naturopathic doctor. We are educated an additional three hundred hours past the typical medical school curriculum in support-ive therapies that do not harm but support all aspects of the patient. This means our toolbox is overflowing with options for treatment. We know that sometimes the textbook treatments don't work. All that means is it is time to shift gears and try something else because in the end, it is what is best for the patient.

In this instance, I reached for ceiba. I had made a stem bark and leaf tincture during a recent trip to Belize. Knowing there was research pertaining to its use for elevated liver enzymes, I decided to add it to our treatment plan. It took about 8 or 12 weeks, but we finally did start to see the liver enzymes go down with continued use. The usual recommendations were milk thistle, yellow dock, burdock, and artichoke, but none of them had done anything. Individual body chemistry between a person and a plant that fits like a key and a lock happens unexpectedly; this is why it's so important to be open to considering a vast range of options.

While kapoks are too big for most residential landscapes, if you've got the space and live in southern or possibly central Florida, this fast-growing tree would be fun to plant. They are such a unique tree visually, and the shade they can provide is amazing. Their creamy white, fragrant blossoms come out in early spring for a showy display. The flowers have 5 stamens fused to a tube at the base. And the fruit! It is cottony fluff (kapok), or like mini clouds that emerge from long green pods.

Ceiba Recipes

INDICATIONS

- Balances blood sugar
- Constipation
- Diabetes, type 2
- Diuretic
- Dizziness
- Fever
- Headaches, tension,
- Hypertension
- Increased sex drive
- Peptic ulcer
- Sore throat
- Wound healing

Generally regarded as safe for all populations. Beware that ceiba can lower blood pressure and blood glucose. If you are on medication for these conditions, consult your healthcare practitioner before using.

SORE THROAT GARGLE

When we treat disorder in the body both locally and systemically, simultaneously, we give the body a huge leg up in the battle. An example is using a neti pot for a sinus infection and also drinking tea of yerba santa, sage, and elderflower. Another example is using a gargle of ceiba while also drinking the tea. Taking good care of ourselves when we're ill is key to recovery. As a society, we love to push through illness, continuing to work or sending our kids to school. While sometimes we don't have the luxury of staying home, as a whole, I think we can do better. Gargling for a sore throat used to be a staple treatment for strep, laryngitis, and pharyngitis but it has become less common although it's effective. This simple approach targets the back of the throat and tonsils, coating them with medicines to fight whatever bacteria or virus is harbored there.

Items needed:
Kettle
16-oz. glass jar
1-oz. jar or jigger
Drinking glass

Ingredients:
2 tbsp. dried ceiba leaves
12 oz. boiling water

Put the leaves into the glass jar and pour the boiling water over them. Cover and let steep for 1 hour. Strain.

Pour 1 oz. into a drinking glass and pour it into the mouth without swallowing. Lean the head back slightly and begin to gargle the infusion. Try to gargle for one minute before spitting out the medicine. Do not eat or drink for 20 minutes afterward. Repeat every 2 to 3 hours until symptoms ease up.

MEDICINAL SLEEP PILLOW

A mature ceiba tree produces hundreds of seed pods each year. Each pod is filled with a soft white, downy cotton that can be harvested and made into medicinal pillows to help various things. I like sleep pillows because the scent and softness are cues for my body to relax and turn off. Like most people, my days vary quite a bit, and I find trying to keep pre-bed sleep rituals constant helps me sleep better and feel more rested in the morning. A sleep pillow is just one piece of that routine.

Items needed:
Pruning shears
Rolling pin
Two mixing bowls
2 4-by-4-inch pieces of cotton fabric
Needle and thread

Ingredients:
20 ceiba seed pods
Essential oil of choice: chamomile, lavender, sandalwood,
      cedarwood, or bergamot

Once you've harvested the kapok pods, line them up and whack each one relatively hard to get the pods to crack open. Pull them apart and remove the cotton from inside.

    Next, separate the cotton from the tiny seeds. This can be tedious, but fun if you make it a group activity. Once the seeds and cotton are separated, sew the two layers of fabric closed on three sides, sewing the fabric inside out if it has a printed pattern. Before stuffing your pillow, add 5 to 15 drops of essential oil (depending on how strong of scent you'd like) to your cotton stuffing and fluff. Turn the pillow right side out and then stuff it with the scented cotton. Stitch up the last side and press the pillow to distribute the filling evenly throughout.

Chestnut

Castanea sativa,
Aesculus
hippocastanum

Family: Fagaceae
and Sapindaceae,
respectively
Parts used: *Castanea
sativa (sweet chest-
nut):* leaves; *Aesculus
hippocastanum (horse
chestnut):* seed, bark
Medicinal actions:
*American Chestnut:
Leaves:* respiratory com-
plaints; *Bark:* diuretic,
emetic, purgative, tonic.
Horse chestnut: antie-
dematous, anti-inflam-
matory, antioxidant, an-
tispasmodic, astringent,
bitter, diuretic, inflam-
matory modulator, tonic,
vascular protective,
vasodilator, venotonic.
Native geography:
Sweet chestnut: western
Asia and southeastern
Europe. *Horse chestnut:*
Balkans

When I was a kid, nuts were a snack only adults ate. They weren't the touted protein snack they are today and, quite honestly, I only ever saw them in bowls at hotel bars and at Christmas. The holiday nut tray was a novelty, with its shiny silver nut-cracker and pick. I was never strong enough to crack the nuts so got I bored of the activity very quickly. But adults seemed to love sitting in our yellow recliner (complete with embroi-dered doily on the back), cracking nuts, and telling stories. One day, I told myself, I *would* be able to crack that chestnut. But I wouldn't just pop it immediately into my mouth, I'd walk it over to the fire and roast it a bit, just like in the song.

At our house the nut tray sat on a wooden end table. This end table was my favorite because it was octagon-shaped and had two panels on the side that opened up like French doors, revealing a large lower compartment. I often hid things there that I didn't want my older brother or sister to find. My candy stash of Sweet Tarts, Tootsie Rolls, and bubble gum, a lipstick stolen from my sister; a lighter of my brother's that was engraved; and sometimes even the cat. It was the most exotic piece of furniture we owned.

I've told my daughter all about the secret treasures I kept in my fancy table. Telling stories was how I got her to cooperate when she was little. The moment I began a new story, her face would brighten, a smile would appear, and she'd quiet down to listen. I would tell her made-up stories based on our family and all of the craziness that united kinships often create. The story of my great-grandad the coal

miner became the centerpiece in epic tales of tunnels and canaries. His granddaughter with the fiery red hair who had had her own adventures after her mama ran away, and my uncle, the luckiest man alive, all featured in tall tales full of mystery. My mother's people come from deep within the Appalachian Trail area in Tennessee. Perhaps that is where my love of storytelling (and chestnuts) began. In front of the home where everyone gathered for noon Sunday dinner grew a giant chestnut tree. It provided nuts to eat and shaded the front porch where we fanned ourselves while drinking iced tea. It also provided endless ammunition for our kid games or for retali-ation when we needed to rectify a perceived injustice.

Like most families, chestnuts themselves are complicated. They aren't like a peanut, where all you have to do is squeeze that flimsy outer shell to reap the reward. They are hard—so hard that even stepping on them rarely cracks the shell. They require real work to reach the prize and the use of specialty, plier-shaped tools. The goal is to crack it equally in half to reveal the two perfect halves inside, or even one unscathed whole nut. But put pressure slightly off-center and you'll crush the meat and feel ridiculously hopeless. And once the shell is off, next comes the delicate, precise work of a surgeon: using a sharp little pick to scrape the nut meat away from the inner pel-licule. At Christmastime, the adult libations often made the grownups lose patience with the whole finicky ordeal, and they'd reach for the nut hammer. With exuberance they would slam the hammer down onto the nut, making

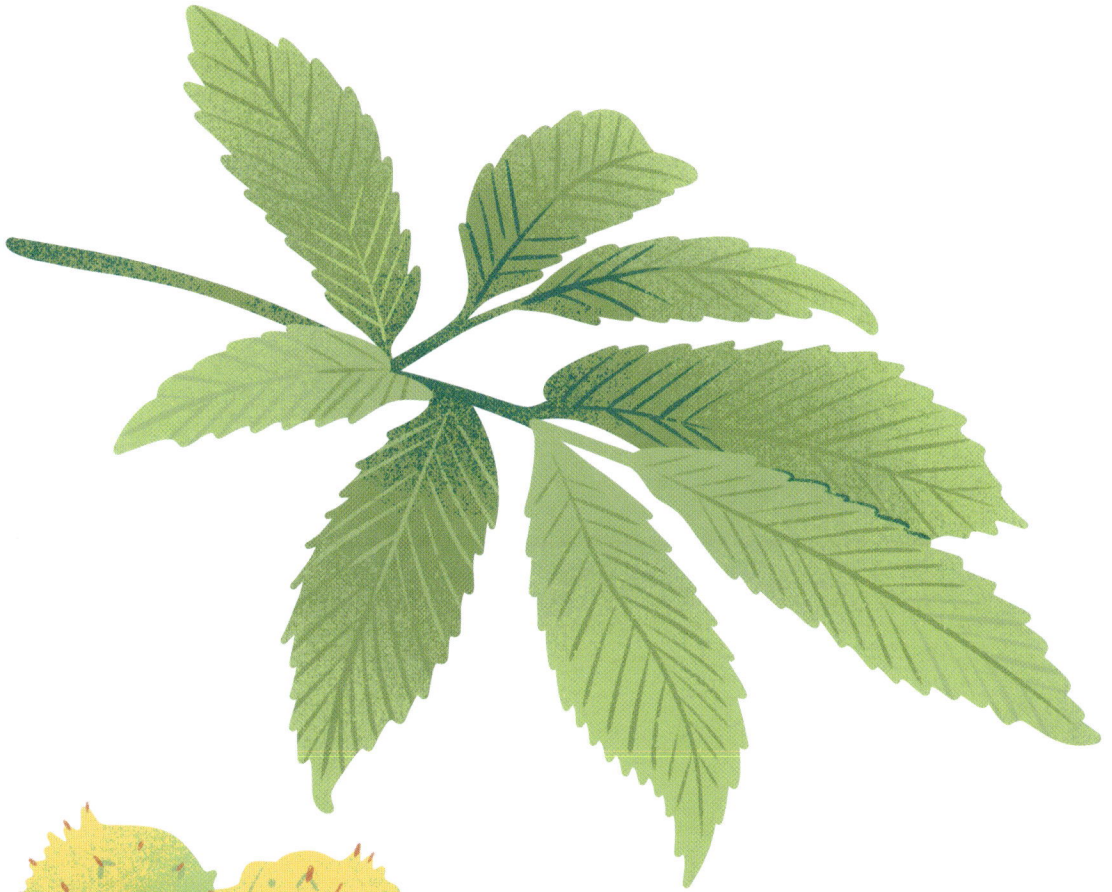

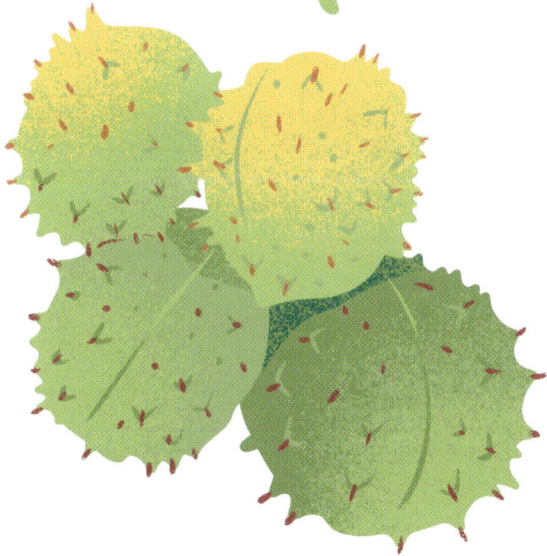

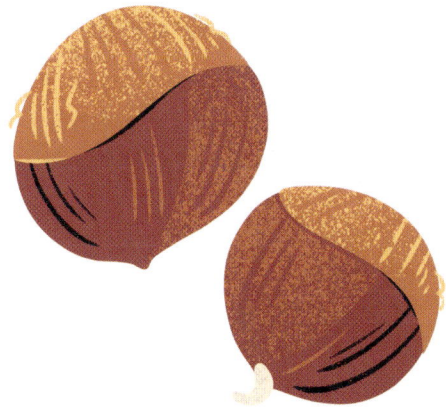

**USDA hardiness
zones:** 3 to 8

Water: average, water
1 to 2 gallons per week
after planting

Light requirement:
sun to part shade

Soil: well-drained,
fertile soil

Temperature:
very cold hardy; should
be pruned in fall

Wildlife notes:
caterpillars of the
triangle moth and horse
chestnut leaf-miner
moth feed on the horse
chestnut leaves. These
caterpillars are a food
source for the blue tit
bird. Many mammals,
including deer, eat the
conkers.

Pollinator friendly:
flowers provide a rich
source of nectar and
pollen for insects

Pests: leaf blotch,
powdery mildew,
anthracnose

its pieces fly all over the place so you had to
shuffle your fingers all over the table to find
bits of the goods.

Perhaps having the nut tray at Christmas
time was a way my mom remembered her
past. Something simple that flooded her mind
with memories. In some similar way, when I
remember our chestnut tree, I think back to
my youth and all of the stories I collected in
its presence, as numerous as the falling nuts
themselves.

———————

While horse chestnuts are usually the species
for sale in botanical shops and referenced in
herbal literature, the leaves and nuts of the
sweet chestnut tree have traditionally been
used as well (and the prolific American chestnut, *Castanea dentata*, before being obliterated
by blight). I've seen occasional mention of the
Cherokee tribes using the chestnut for a multitude of things, such as lumber, dye, food, and
firewood, and surely many Native American
tribes living in the hardwood forests of eastern North America would have also used them
when they formed such a large component of
the native forests. As far as a medicinal use,
it is referenced that it was used for stomach
pains and typhoid.

Culpeper's Complete Herbal and the
U.S. Pharmacopoeia (1873–1905) listed
the chestnut when a strong astringent was
needed. Astringents pull tissues together
and often reduce or stop fluid flow, so this
would indicate diarrhea, excessive menstrual
bleeding, postpartum bleeding, or bleeding
from a wound. Dried mature leaves were also
used to form astringent compounds. This is
most likely due to their relatively high tannin
levels. The ground nuts were used as a poultice
for treating toothaches, and the spring leaves
were used topically for burns, joint pains,

sores, and swellings. The leaves were used
for upper respiratory colds, coughs, and sore
throats.

Today horse chestnuts are most commonly available, and I use them as a herbal
remedy anytime a circulatory or venous
issue arises. Horse chestnut shines when it
comes to alleviating congestion or improving insufficiency of the venous system—the
massive and intricate network of veins. These
veins traverse your entire body, weaving and
connecting blood vessels and organ systems
like a super speed highway. Deoxygenated
blood—blood that has traveled from the heart
and lungs and dropped off its oxygen load—
travels along this highway back to the heart/
lung hub to pick up another oxygen load.
Imagine a circle. At the top is the heart and
lungs and oxygenated blood. From the top to
the halfway point is the artery highway, which
is filled with oxygenated traffic. At the halfway
point, the oxygen gets dumped and the venous
system is the second half of the circle back up
to the top.

These highways can get backed up with
traffic and sometimes even require detours
due to venous integrity (or lack thereof).
Because the system includes both large vessels
and the tiniest of capillaries, it can be challenging to keep all the roads open, so to speak.
Horse chestnut creates selective vascular
permeabilization. What this means is that
if part of the venous system is injured or weakened, the body releases a signal. As a result the
calcium channels, the doorways into the cells,
become sensitive to healing ions, which result
in increased venous tone. Tone is a good thing.
Tone = venous strength and proper function.

I don't like to play favorites, but when
I see the late spring bloom of the horse
chestnut, it definitely bestills my heart. A
Horse chestnut bloom is very distinct with its
cone shaped stacked flowers. They are mostly

creamy in color but pinkish at the base and seem to explode onto the tree suddenly in late spring. As pollinators move towards their busiest time of year they quickly ascend onto the Horse chestnut. After pollination and as the flower dies, they turn into a glossy red-brown conker inside a spiky green husk, which will fall before winter.

Chestnut Recipes

INDICATIONS

- Backache
- Bruising
- Cellulite
- Circulatory stimulant and tonic
- Cold hands and feet
- Deep leg thrombosis
- Edema
- Hemorrhoids
- Spider veins
- Varicose veins
- Venous value tonic

*The following information is regarding horse chestnut. Raw nuts are toxic. Avoid if diagnosed with bleeding disorders as horse chestnut may affect platelet aggregation. Avoid if pregnant and/or breastfeeding.

GUT BALLS

One of my favorite ways to combat a bout of constipation is with something I call "gut balls." I realize that's a terrible name. When I made my first batch I was beginning to hit a creativity wall from operating three herb shops while still seeing patients. But the name stuck with my kids, so at some point there was no turning back. When treating constipation, my motto is "go easy." No one needs to have a traumatic release after things have built up for a while. Eating your medicine helps to target the herbs right where you need them—in this case, the colon.

Items needed:
Mixing bowl
Mixing spoon
Airtight container

Ingredients:
1 oz. horse chestnut powder
½ oz. ground flaxseed
½ oz. marshmallow powder
⅛ oz. licorice root powder
½ oz. cacao powder
¼ to ½ cup of honey
¼ c to 1 cup nut butter of choice (optional)

Mix all dry ingredients in a bowl, then add the honey and nut butter. Roll into 1-inch balls **and keep in an airtight container in the refrigerator for up to two weeks.**

ROASTED CHESTNUTS

With a high content of vitamin C and antioxidants, chestnuts are a valuable addition to the winter diet when colds and flus are swirling around. They also contain gallic and ellagic acid, powerful antioxidants that are actually concentrated after cooking. Learning how to roast and add chestnuts to your wintry dishes can really give you an immune boost as well as a satisfying meal. One of my go-tos is a Japanese dish called *kuri gohan*, translated as "chestnut rice." It's warm and savory, but you can adjust the flavors much like a congee recipe and make it sweet if you wish. Roasting chestnuts isn't necessarily easy, but worth the trouble. I suggest setting aside some designated time to the task when you can slow down and relax into the process.

Items needed:
Stockpot
Strainer
Paring knife
Bowl

Ingredients:
15 to 20 horse chestnuts
2 cups short-grain rice
2 tbsp. mirin
1 tbsp. sake
1 tsp. bonito flakes
½ tsp. salt
Black sesame seeds, toasted

Bring a stockpot of water to a boil and then add chestnuts. The purpose of boiling the chestnuts is to soften the outer skin, which makes them easier to peel and clean.

After three minutes, strain the nuts and begin removing the outer peel and the inner skin. You want to do this while they are still warm as the heat softens the peel. Using a paring knife, cut around the base of the nut and begin to peel upward. Once the peel is removed, gently use the knife to clean out the nut and remove any inner peel from the crevices. Give the nuts one more rinse and set them aside.

Using a rice cooker or a stovetop pan, cook the rice. Once the rice is ready, stir in the mirin, sake, bonito flakes, and salt. Close the lid again and let it rest for 30 minutes. A rice cooker makes it easier to maintain the heat here, but a pot will also do the job. After 30 minutes, scoop some into a bowl and top each serving with 4 or 5 chestnuts.

Crab Apple

Malus sylvestris

Family: Rosaceae
Parts used: fruit, leaves, flowers, bark
Medicinal actions: anti-inflammatory, antioxidant, aperient, bitter, febrifuge, laxative, tonic
Native geography: Europe, Asia, Africa; in the US they can now be found in the Midwest, Mid-Atlantic, and most of the South, as well as the Northeast

I grew up in Lincoln, Nebraska. While we didn't have apple trees there, our driveway was lined with crab apples, trees that produce tiny little sour apples that are rarely appreciated anymore but were once highly valued.

Our house had a hole in the hallway floor on the second story that acted as a laundry chute. We'd lift up the orange shag carpet to reveal a metal chute—*bombs away*, we sent our laundry straight to the basement, where the washer and dryer were. With three kids in the house, of course many other things slid down that laundry chute—and sometimes came up it, too. When my older brother Reese wanted to play with me, he'd turn up the song "Kung Fu Fighting" in his basement bedroom and the refrain would drift up the laundry chute. It was our signal.

His bedroom was in the basement for two reasons. One, because he'd seen a ghost on the attic stairs once and had decided then and there that his bedroom should be as far away as possible from that attic. And two, he had a waterbed. In the 1970s, waterbeds were the end all, be all of coolness. It was like lying on a raft in the middle of a swimming pool, all night. Even as someone who doesn't have a particular affinity for water, I still thought it was amazing. I'd crawl to the center of the bed and log roll from one side to the other, listening to the water sloshing all around me.

Reese was the coolest guy I knew. Eight years older than me and the only sibling that actually paid attention to me, he demonstrated love in a way no one else did in the family, and I cherished every second I could get. He had a whole big life I could hardly understand, but while he was still living in the same house, he found small ways to acknowledge me. Secret glances that made me feel special, like we had a running inside joke. When my dad's hackles got up, Reese would give me a side eye to reassure me that it would blow over.

One night I got to go to Reese's high school. It was his senior year. I watched him in a play called 1984. The plot was way over my head, but it didn't matter because I was watching my idol doing something so brave, and doing it really well. In my mind, Reese could do anything. I don't believe there is a single childhood photo of Reese where he is just smiling at the camera. He is always striking a pose, making a face to turn the opportunity into a moment.

His friends used to come over and play basketball in our long, fairly narrow driveway. Our house was to one side, and a row of crab apple trees lined the other. The trees were technically in the neighbors' yard, but the majority of the branches hung over our driveway as they reached for the sun. I can still see my brother out there, with those trees as a backdrop, all bare and scraggly in the winter as he shoveled the snow so we could get the car out and onto the slippery streets. And in the spring, with their brilliant dark pink blossoms and in the summer, with their bright green and shimmery leaves. And of course in the fall, when all of us were assigned to scrape and clean the driveway of the fallen fruit. We kids loved to splatter and squish them with our shoes and throw them at one another to see if we could get them to explode

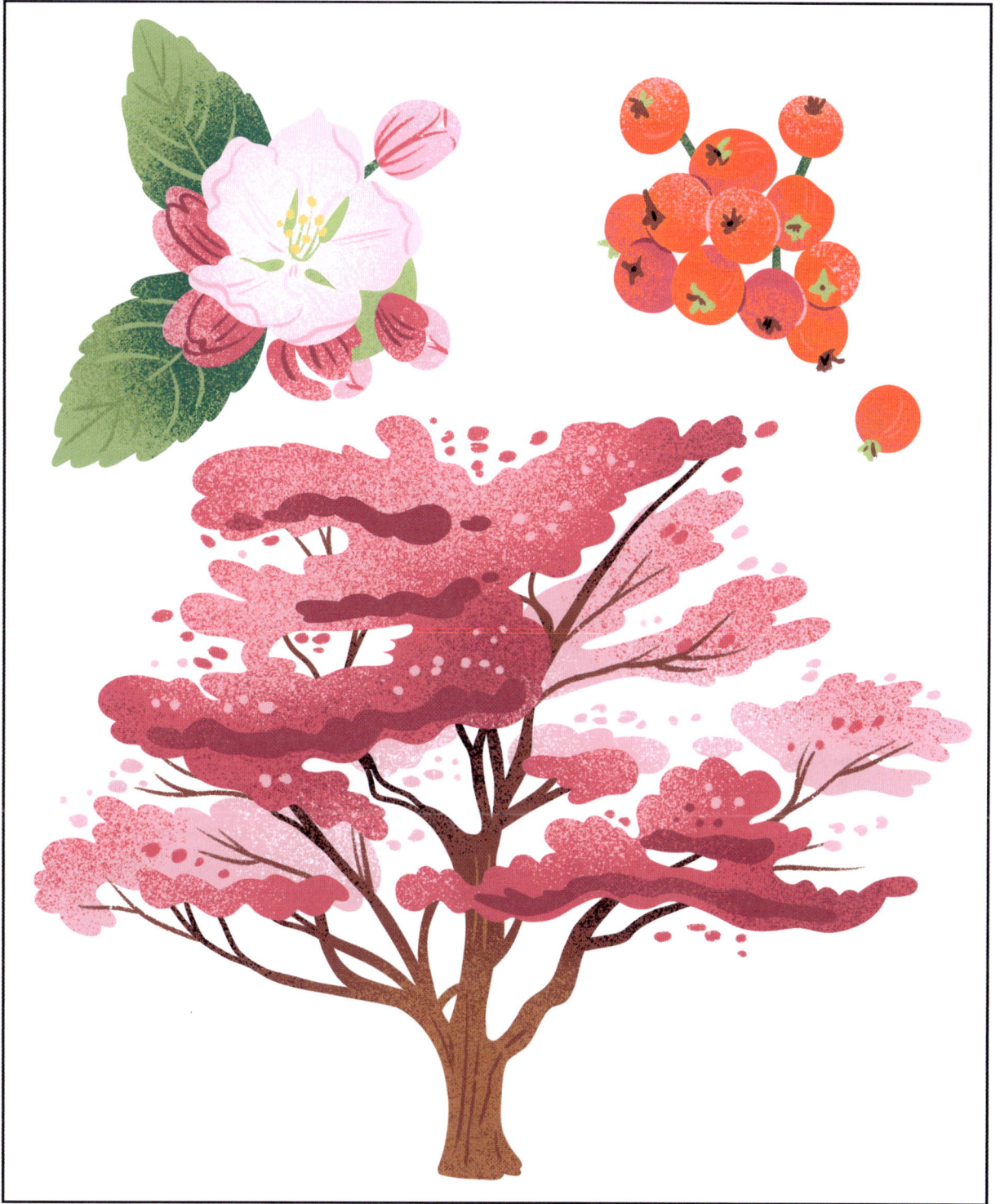

**USDA hardiness
zones:** 4 to 8
Water: need abundant moisture during their vegetative period, but prefer much less moisture in winter
Light requirement: part shade
Soil: moist and well drained, well limed
Temperature: intolerant of frost
Wildlife notes: loved by many bird varieties, rabbits, squirrels, opossums, raccoons, skunks, and foxes
Pollinator friendly: supports spring bees
Pests: cedar apple rust, fire blight, apple scab

as they hit. The crab apples were the bane of my mom's existence in fall, since flies would descend thickly on the decomposing fruit. But then, the following spring it was like she had amnesia—she'd inevitably rave about the glorious beauty of those blossoms. And they do put on quite a display. They grow up to 40 feet tall, with almost as much spread, and they tend to blossom heavily in snowy clumps. The true wild apple blooms in spring, but new cultivars can bloom at various times. They produce lovely, fragrant white or pink blossoms, typically with 5 petals.

The last time I saw Reese, we met up in Brooklyn, New York. We watched my daughter play on the playground. He loved children; I'll always feel sad that he never got to be a dad. Even then, he still talked to me as a younger sister with wise big-brother energy. We shared our love of sushi, talked about angel numbers, traveling, and random memories of our family. The entire time I kept looking at this tree across from us, and it wasn't until I got home and looked it up that I realized that it was also a crab apple.

Crab apple has a long history in herbal folk medicine. For centuries, medicinal knowledge was passed from one generation to the next. At the heart of this knowledge was how to find, collect, and use plants to heal the ailments of the family. Not only was this information key for survival, but it instilled a strength, a confidence that people could, to some degree, take care of themselves. Crab apple used to be called "wild apple" because it was found in the forests. While a bit bitter as a raw fruit, it makes great jellies, jams, and pie. It was also foraged to use as a soothing and moistening sore throat treatment.

Because the flesh of the fruit produces a cooling effect, the fruit can also be mashed and spread onto the skin in the case of burns and insect bites to provide relief. You can also mix the mashed fruit with the leaves to create a natural antibacterial wound treatment, as the leaves contain up to 2.4% of an antibacterial substance called florin.

The bitter principle of crab apple (what you taste when you bite into one) has a few different effects. Bitter compounds are recognized for stimulating digestion. By consuming a bit of crab apple at the beginning of a meal it can, in the same way an aperitif does, initiate the digestive process. This prompts the stomach to create hydrochloric acid (HCL), which is necessary for proper digestive function. It also promotes positive bowel movements. When I say "positive" what I'm implying is that crab apple can help move stool along without the harsh side effects caused by many laxatives. Crab apple extract has also been used against parasites, once again due to the bitter and possibly the phenolic compounds.

Throughout medicinal literature, crab apple is recommended for reducing fevers and cooling inflammations. It is even listed in the tenth-century Anglo-Saxon anthology

Lacnunga [Remedies] as one of the "nine herb charms" used for illness and infection. While crab apple seems has been somewhat neglected in modern herbal practice, I suggest not discounting it. All healing plants have inherent value if employed at the right time and place.

Crab apples are ready for harvest in late summer or early fall. Most fruits range between 1 to 2 inches in size. Slice them up and dehydrate the fruit for later use, pulverize the dehydrated bits into powder, or make an herbal tincture. Just don't forget to save a few for some jam or a late-summer pie.

Crab Apple Recipes

INDICATIONS

- Appetite stimulant
- Blood sugar regulation
- Burns
- Constipation
- Cystitis
- Diarrhea
- Digestive regulator
- Fevers
- Gout
- Insect bites
- Parasite eradication
- Sore throat
- Wound healing

Raw seeds are toxic. Eating raw crab apples in excess can cause stomach cramps.

CRAB APPLE JAM

Turning medicine into food is one of my favorite things. If I can incorporate herbs into my daily life without having to remember to drink this tea or take that capsule, it is a win. Almost any herb that contains a medicinal fruit can be turned into a jelly or a jam—morning toast can become a nutritional, medicinal treat. This recipe is not only supportive for the digestive system, but with the added hawthorn and raspberries, you have both an antioxidant boost and heart tonic.

Making jam is much easier than most people think. Unlike vegetables, you don't have to pressure cook or boil jam for long periods of time. You can collect crab apples in the morning and have jam by lunchtime.

Because crab apples aren't uniform in size, any harvest will yield slightly different volumes of pulp. Be sure to follow the insert guide included with your pectin to determine the correct amount to add for your batch.

Items needed:
2 Stockpots
Saucepan
Mixing bowl
6 16-oz. glass canning jars
Canning tongs
Canning funnel

Ingredients:
2 lbs. crab apples
8 oz. dried rose hips
½ lb. fresh hawthorn berry
5 oz. raspberries
Pomona's low-sugar pectin

First, rehydrate the rose hips. Put them into a saucepan and add enough water to cover them. Bring it to a simmer, turn off the heat, and then let them sit for one hour. Strain.

Mix the sugar and pectin together in a bowl and set aside.

Next, fill up a stock pot with water and set to boil. Once boiling, add your 6 jars and boil them for 10 minutes to sanitize them. Pull them out carefully with canning tongs and set them upside down on a clean dish towel. Keep the stockpot water simmering in the meantime.

Put the crab apples, rose hips, and hawthorn berries into a different stockpot and gently warm them to soften up the fruits. Be careful not to cook them completely, however—add a touch of water if needed. Once they are soft, turn off the heat, add the raspberries and mash completely. Next, add calcium water as directed by the pectin package and turn the heat on to medium.

Slowly begin to add the sugar/pectin mixture into the fruit in the stock pot, stirring continuously. Bring to a boil and boil for 1 minute before removing it from the heat. Skim off any foam that coats the surface, then ladle the jam into jars. The jars should still be warm at the time of filling. Put the tops on and put them into the stockpot with hot water. The jars should be completely submerged in boiling water for 10 minutes.

Remove with canning tongs and set on a towel to cool. Be sure to label and date the jars.

Dogwood

Cornus nuttallii,
Cornus kousa

Family: Cornaceae
Parts used: bark, flower
Medicinal actions:
antiperiodic, astringent,
cathartic, febrifuge,
laxative, stimulant,
and tonic
Native geography:
Cornus nuttallii: western
North America from
British Columbia to
California, New York,
and North Carolina.
Cornus kousa: Japan,
China, Korea

They call her Queen of the Forest. My first herbal mentor, Linda Quintana, used to walk me around her big, beautiful herb garden, pouring out copious amounts of information that I desperately tried to scribble down in my notebook. One day, she insisted I put the notebook down. She wanted me to take everything in more intuitively as we meandered down paths and in and out of garden beds. We did this once a week; she exchanged knowledge for gardening help. Our sessions always ended with a plant meditation. This involved me doing my best to follow my intuition and selecting a particular plant that was "speaking" to me that day. I would set my little mat down close by the plant I had chosen and do my best to meditate. Over time, it got easier. The idea was to try to listen to what the plant had to say.

The funny thing was, most times, what I thought I'd "heard" in my meditations turned out to be the same information that I would later read in my herbal medicine books. My process was this: I would work in the garden, learning from Linda throughout the day, and before heading home I would do my meditation. Then I would go home, write in my journal what I'd gathered from my meditation, and then grab my herb books and read up on the plant. At first I thought it was a fluke, but it kept happening, week after week.

Dogwood often came into my mind when I would meditate. There is a relationship that grows when you are invested in studying herbal medicine. As with most relationships, it begins with genuine enthusiasm. There is a joy that you can feel when you participate in your first herb walk or herbal conference. I often say this is an ancient knowledge, embedded deep within a cellular level that suddenly awakens. Similar to when a gene turns on or off with epigenetics, the DNA that has held this knowledge for generations gets turned back on. We all naturally want to be able to care for ourselves and those around us—for centuries, herbs have helped us do that.

This led to me developing a personal motto: you can read about herbs all day long, but until you sit with them, you really don't know much at all. You need to smell them, taste them, and feel what they do inside your own body. Herbs are classified in different ways, including bitter, sweet, and slick, but the experience of working with them yourself is how you truly learn herbal medicine. This was how I truly got to know dogwood in a wild and rugged forest in Arkansas.

Although it was a warm spring day, I felt cold whenever the sun dipped behind the clouds. I wrapped my sweater around my chest tightly and went stomping into the woods on a new trail I'd discovered on an old map. A trail that wasn't overly developed like in so many state parks. Brown was still the dominant color, but green was poking out everywhere and it was obvious it would soon overtake the color palette. I came to a clearing and, almost like a fairy tale, there stood the most perfect light pink dogwood I'd ever seen. When dogwoods are in full bloom there is something magical and mythical about them, the unicorn of the forest. I had a sudden urge to sit beneath its branches and settle up

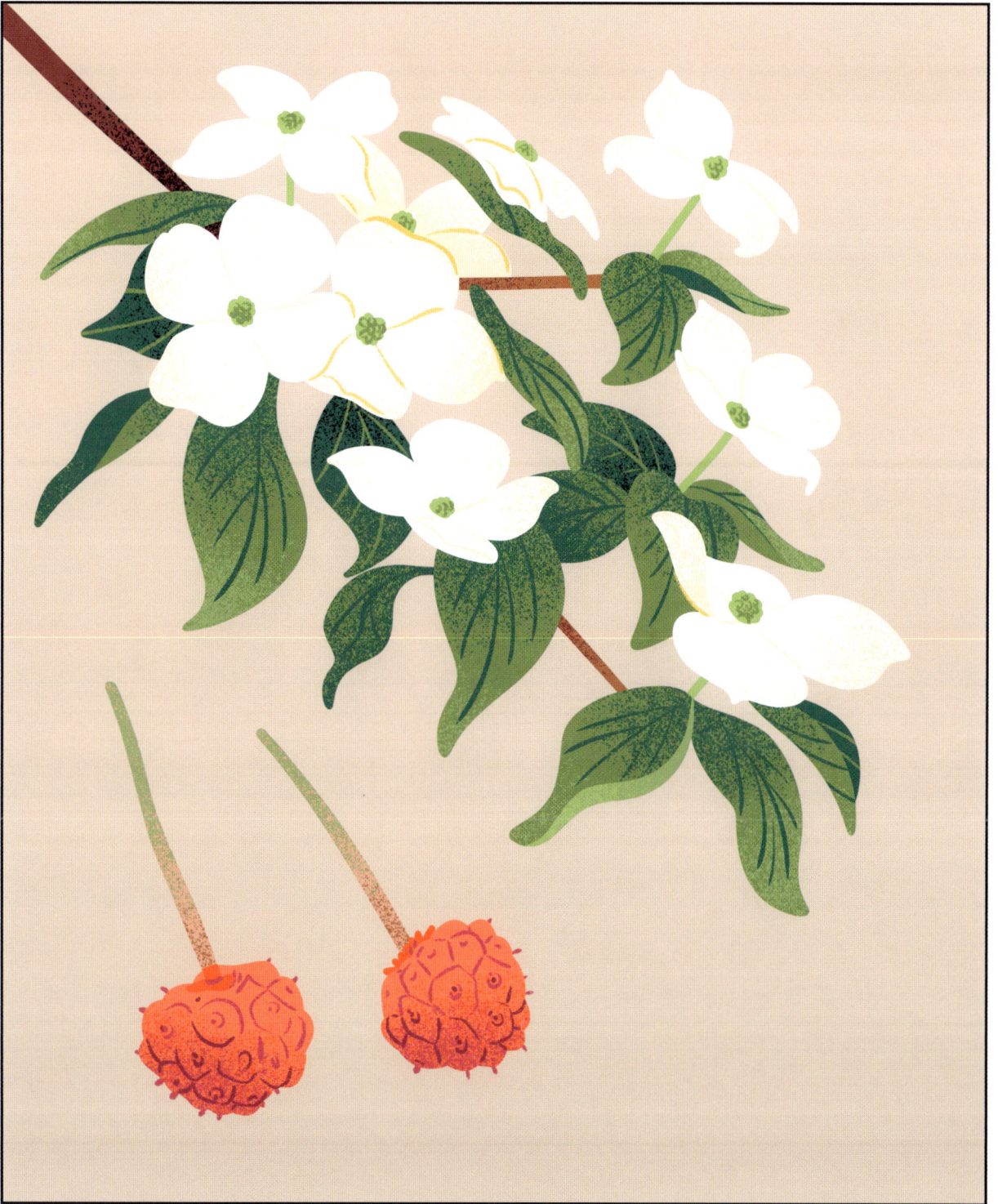

USDA hardiness zones: 7 to 9

Water: if rainfall is insufficient, water enough to soak several inches into the soil once a week

Light requirement: part shade; bark damaged by hot sun

Soil: well-drained acid soils high in organic matter

Temperature: cold hardy, but temperature swings in spring can cause stress which may result in in fewer flowers

Wildlife notes: Deer and elk like the leaves; many small mammals and birds eat the fruit, particularly band-tailed pigeons and pileated woodpeckers

Pollinator friendly: attracts the azure butterfly

Pests: anthracnose, powdery mildew, dogwood borer, dogwood club-gall midge

against it with my back on its thin trunk. I opened my backpack to pull out a thermos of hot water I had with me, added a handful of dogwood blossoms, and let it steep for a few minutes. After pouring myself a cup of tea, I began my plant meditation ritual. I inhaled deeply to smell the steam wafting up from the cup, and I let the thoughts it elicited roll through my brain. Slowly bringing it to my lips, I filled my mouth and held it there before swallowing the floral bouquet. I recognized a slightly warming quality to the tea and felt its energy settle in the middle of my back. After taking a few more sips, I got out my notebook and wrote down all the thoughts I'd just experienced. Some made sense, others seemed random, but I never filter my journaling experience. I pressed a couple of the blossoms in my book, gave gratitude to the dogwood, and walked myself out of the woods. I was ready to go home and read all about it.

———————

A spring-blooming dogwood is one of life's simple pleasures. They can be easily cultivated and with proper pruning and care can fit in almost any landscape. The leaves bud out in spring once temperatures consistently reach 55° F. At first they don't look like much, just a slight extension of the branch stem. They appear opposite on ½ inch petioles with blades that are ovate-elliptic and taper to a point. If you look underneath the leaf, you'll see and feel soft little hairs growing there. And while the flowers steal the show in spring, the leaves do produce a nice fall display along with bright red-orange fruit.

A few years ago, I had to make the unfortunate decision of whether to remove my gallbladder. A polyp had been detected on a routine ultrasound, and while it wasn't quite big enough to be labeled a concern yet, it was

close. As someone who tries to avoid invasive medical treatments unless they're absolutely necessary, I hemmed and hawed about this for quite some time. The thought of losing a whole organ seemed concerning, especially one that plays such a part in healthy digestion. On the other hand, I would always worry that the polyp was there.

In the end I decided to have it removed. There probably isn't a right or wrong here, but my biggest concern was how to rebalance my digestive process in the absence of my gallbladder. The liver produces bile, which breaks down dietary fats into fatty acids; the gallbladder stores it. Some fatty acids are beneficial for the body, such as olive oil and fish. Others, like trans fats (from fried food, or processed foods) can hurt the body in many different ways. Without a gallbladder, your body will still have access to bile as the liver makes it, but there isn't a stockpile ready to go. If you are eating a relatively balanced diet, that typically is okay. But what about when you eat a marbled steak or something else with a higher fat ratio?

This is when I reach for dogwood. The bitter principle in the bark and flowers stimulate bile from the liver to move into the small intestine, specifically the duodenum. The duodenum is where food and liquid goes after leaving the stomach. This is a crucial stopping point in digestion. The food, liquid, bile, and digestive enzymes from the pancreas all meet here and get to work to determine what should be absorbed as valuable nutrition and what excreted. The former continues on down the track for eventual reabsorption; the latter heads to the waste department (the large intestines and kidneys).

Many Pacific Northwest tribes also used *Cornus nuttallii* as a digestive aid and blood purifier. Herbalists call the blood-purifying action an "alterative," which is defined as an herb that produces gradual beneficial change in the body, usually by improving nutrition. We can infer, then, that an improved digestion process is one that leads to increased nutritional uptake from the foods we eat. This results in improved mental function, increased energy, and better physical performance.

Dogwood Recipes

INDICATIONS

- Acne
- Bile regulation
- Body aches and pains
- Constipation
- Digestive tonic
- Eczema
- Intermittent Fever
- Headaches
- Malaria
- Stress from repressed emotion

Due to aspirin-like salicylates in dogwood, a percentage of the population might experience stomach irritation after taking.

DOGWOOD MUFFINS

Cornus nuttallii is typically what you'll encounter in a medicinal tincture, but the fruit that the *Cornus kousa* produces has endless potential. They are easily collected in the late summer and early fall. These little fruits are packed with powerful antioxidants and are known to support liver detoxification and increase energy levels. Mix up a batch of these muffins for a healthy addition to any breakfast.

Items needed:
Oven, preheated to 400° F
12-cup muffin tin
2 mixing bowls
Food mill

Ingredients:
2 cups of all-purpose flour
2 tsp. baking powder
1 tsp. baking soda
1 tsp. salt
1 ½ cups kousa dogwood berry purée
⅔ cup light brown sugar
⅔ cup unsalted butter, melted
1 large egg
1 tsp. vanilla extract
Sliced almonds and raw cane sugar to sprinkle on top of the muffins

Making the purée is the first step, and having a food mill is the easiest way to accomplish this. The food mill removes the skin, seeds, and pulp while creating purée at the same time. Make the purée, set aside.

Combine flour, baking powder, baking soda, and salt together in the mixing bowl. Set aside.

In a different bowl, whisk together the purée, sugar, butter, egg, and vanilla extract. Gently fold in your flour blend, just until mixed. Do not over stir.

In a greased muffin tin, scoop out the batter and divide evenly. Sprinkle each muffin compartment with sliced almonds and a touch of sugar.

Bake for 20 to 25 minutes. Cool before removing from the pan.

APERITIF FOR DIGESTION

Using *Cornus nuttallii* to stimulate the digestive system before meals can help process food efficiently and reduce gut inflammation. Just a touch is needed to trigger the bitter response, which wakes up the stomach and alerts the lower digestive tract. With so many of us eating on the go, we are losing the important bodily cues needed to spark digestion. Without them, we don't have the necessary enzymes pumping needed to break down our food. A dose of dogwood aperitif revs the system to be ready to go.

Items needed:
Mason jar
Wax paper
Rubber band

Ingredients:
¼ cup *Cornus nuttallii* bark
½ cup apple cider vinegar

Add the bark to the mason jar and cover it with apple cider vinegar. Cut a square of wax paper to put over the top, and secure it with a rubber band. Then put on the mason jar lid, both top and screw band. The wax paper protects the lid from the vinegar, but you still need the lid affixed so you can shake the jar without making a mess.

Store in a cool, dark place for two weeks, shaking vigorously daily.

Strain and store in a dropper bottle. Be sure to label with the date and contents.

Take 2 dropperfuls before each meal.

Douglas Fir

Pseudotsuga menziesii

Family: Pinaceae
Parts used: bark, root, needle, pitch, essential oil
Medicinal actions: Antibacterial, anti-inflammatory, antimicrobial, antispasmodic, carminative, diuretic, expectorant, tonic, vulnerary
Native geography: western North America from Mexico to the Canadian Rockies, from sea level to mountains. Now widely planted as a forestry timber tree.

My husband and I were all set to purchase a different piece of property, a different house. But I kept dreaming about the Douglas fir trees on some land we had previously considered. Big, beautiful Douglas firs. Probably fifty in all and all of them over one hundred feet tall. They perch themselves in a longitudinal grove along the north side of the property, just behind a bluff that leads up to the house. They offer a deep dark green screen, all year round. In the winter the great horned owls return, and I can hear them through the fog, calling back and forth. In the spring robins busily build nests in them—we know the babies are born when we see the remnants of the cracked blue eggs on the ground beneath the trees. The stellar jays use them for their covert operations of diving and squawking at any cats that walk below. The tops of the trees, however, are reserved for the hawks, crows, and the occasional eagle. But twice a year, during migration, we get thousands of birds passing through on their way north or south. There are so many (17.6 million in 2024) that it has been named the Pacific Flyway. We receive alerts on our phone that remind us to turn off all outside lights at night to make it easier for the birds to navigate. It is a short-lived biannual experience but the sudden burst of bird noise that erupts on our farm lets us know when it's in full swing. When these travelers descend onto our Douglas fir trees, it is like an international airport with all of them talking at once about the long journey, the day's events, and taking roll call to make sure everyone in their tribe made the flight. The kids and I, and a couple of our farm cats, all sit outside in wonder and listen to their songs, chatter, and calls. It's a blissful seasonal mark.

In various shamanic and Indigenous traditions, north represents wisdom and is often associated with the elders in a family or culture. I view the Doug firs on our property as elders, too. These trees that have witnessed and recorded the events happening on this land over the last two hundred years. They lived here when the Atfalati occupied this land. I view these trees as protectors, hugging the house and all of us in it with a gentle embrace. The elders are also the ones who possess stories, and I often walk among these trees listening for any wisdom they might wish to share. I wonder how many hands have touched them, how many souls have found respite in their shade.

The two biggest trees on the property are in our backyard, on top of a little berm. The trunks of these trees are both 11 feet in circumference—if I and both of my children hold hands, we can just reach all the way around. These trees are twins, melded as one at the base. In most tree pairs, usually one of the two trunks is smaller, but not so with ours. There is a little spot you can step through just where the trunks begin to split. I have vivid memories of my children hopping through this magical "tree door," their hands pressed against the rough bark on either side to brace themselves. They'd jump through and run onto a nearby rope swing held in place by a grandfather branch. Their hair flying behind them, they'd giggle and swing up to the heavens. These trees' branches

MEDICINE FROM THE TREES

80

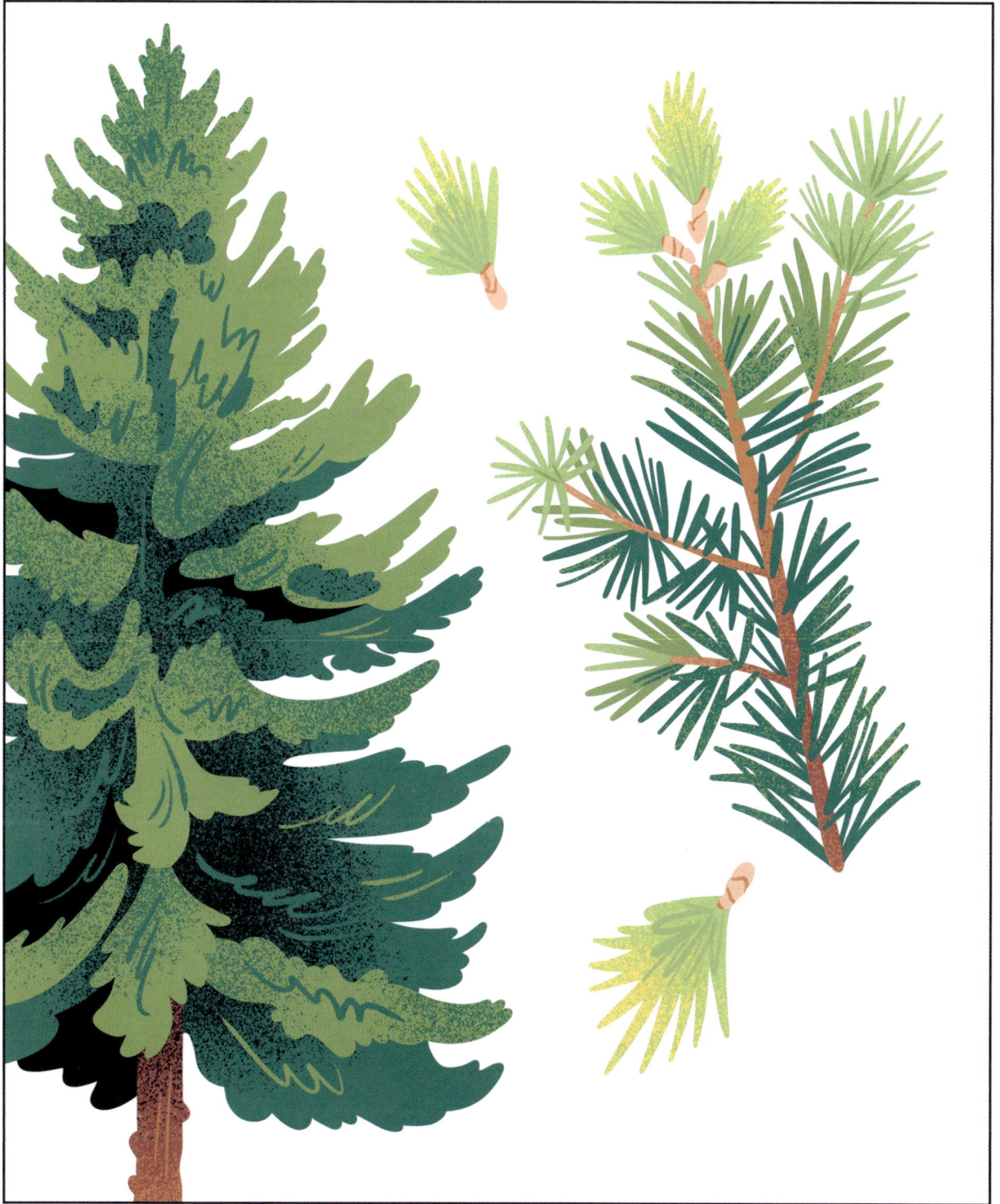

**USDA hardiness
zones:** 3 to 6 (but I live
in 8 and they grow well)
Water: moderate sum-
mer watering for newly
established trees; once
established water needs
are minimal
Light requirement:
full sun to partial shade
Soil: neutral to slightly
acidic, moist, well-
drained soil; does not
grow well in chalky or
boggy soils
Temperature: hardy
to -20°F
Wildlife notes: the
northern spotted owl
and the marbled mur-
relet live in Douglas firs
Pollinator friendly:
carpenter bees collect
its sap; hosts some
species of butterfly
Pests: Douglas fir beetle
and large pin weevil,
dark honey fungus

swoop down toward the south, always toward
the light, and their needles grow in fluffy
bunches that overlap. This creates a canopy
of dry play space year round—I also stop
there as a midway shelter between the house
and the goat barn when it's raining.

Our biggest storms usually happen in late
fall and winter, and I watch these tree giants
twist and blow in the wind. It is as if their
branches dance with the weather, gracefully
releasing all that no longer serves them, like
a dog who shakes the water off after a bath. I
often wish I could shake things off as easily.
Their branches shake and swirl with the wind
gusts and I envision them pulling in water and
carbon dioxide much like we pull in oxygen.
I'll walk around the yard afterward and find the
branches and little limbs that have freed themselves and floated to the ground. When I look
up, it seems as though the entire tree is breathing more fully. It is at this point I can hear my
elders whispering in my ear and encouraging
me to pause, remember to breathe.

————

The Douglas fir—although not actually a fir
tree, nor a true pine—represents a complete
medicine cabinet all in one tree. These trees
are so common in the Pacific Northwest they
are often overlooked at garden centers as an
option for landscaping. People often gravitate
to a species that offers some kind of show:
Does it have a big spring bloom or fall color
display? I wish I could tell every shopper
about their movement. There are few trees that
move in the wind like a Douglas fir. I could
watch them endlessly.

This tall and stately tree needs plenty of
room. It grows slowly, so planting seedlings
will be an act taken for the benefit of future
generations. In spring, bright green needle
shoots appear and can be harvested from

spring to midsummer. Harvest mature needles at any time. One study showed a signifi-
cant increase in terpene concentration from
mid-June to early August. Bark and pitch can
be harvested year-round and dried for later
use. The tree does produce seeds, but only
after ten years.

Bioregional medicine is a term used to
describe medicine derived from the plants
in your local area. It is also how we explain
why particular plants that grow in specific
regions aid in healing the common illnesses
of that region. For example, here in the Pacific
Northwest, where the winters are damp and
chilly, people often contract respiratory colds
that present as damp. Dampness in the lungs
looks like copious amounts of phlegm, often
difficult to expel from the lungs. Luckily,
Douglas fir is an excellent eradicator of dampness in the body. Simply steaming the needles
in hot water releases the aromatics from
the leaves, and you now have a two-in-one
treatment. By breathing in the vapor from the
infusion, you inhale part of the medicine. And
by drinking the infusion, you draw it deeper
into the body for even more healing.

The next time you walk around your lawn,
or in the woods close by, take an account of
what plants are growing of their own accord.
Maybe you'll see dandelions, yellow dock, or
plantain—all valuable medicines at the ready
for common ailments you might encounter.
Douglas fir has a long history of use as support for the immune system and the respiratory tract, to aid digestive complaints, soothe
bladder ailments, and heal skin wounds and
irritations. While most of these applications
originate from the oral histories of the First
Nations, modern research reinforces why
Douglas fir was successful with these cases.
Douglas fir is antimicrobial and antibacterial.
It has the ability to wipe out a wide range of
bacteria and fungi. This, combined with its

antioxidant properties, make it an excellent choice for conditions like bladder cystitis, bronchitis, and infected wounds. Interestingly enough, the needles are also high in vitamin C, always a great addition whenever we need to raise the bar on immune function.

Douglas Fir Recipes

————

INDICATIONS

- Bladder complaints
- Bronchitis
- Colds
- Cough
- Diarrhea
- Intestinal bleeding
- Joint pain
- Mouthwash
- Sinusitis
- Vitamin C
- Wound healing

Generally regarded as safe for all populations. Be aware that Douglas fir can look very similar to Western or Pacific Yew tree.

DOUGLAS FIR SHOWER BOMBS

For me, finding time to shower is a luxury, so I often try to turn that time into a mini self-care session to escape from the daily to-dos and constant bombardment of requests. One of my favorite spa-like additions is a shower bomb. At times they are used for a specific purpose, such as helping to clear up nasal congestion or to alleviate stress. Other times they're just to fill the steam with a pleasant aroma. Douglas fir shower bombs instantly transport me to the forest with their pine-y, woodsy scent.

Items needed:
2 mixing bowls
Mixer, either stand or handheld
Silicone mold of choice, or you can hand-roll

Ingredients:
2 cups baking soda
½ cup citric acid (optional, but it keeps your bomb from crumbling)
20 drops of Douglas fir essential oil,
    or ¼ cup of spring Douglas fir tips, ground
1½ tbsp. water

Combine the baking soda and citric acid in the bowl of the mixer on its lowest setting and blend for 10 seconds.

In a separate bowl, combine the water and the Douglas fir (either essential oil or ground tips).

Turn the mixer on its lowest setting and slowly add the water/Douglas fir mixture just until all ingredients are just blended.

Hand-roll the mixture into 1-inch patties or press into a silicone mold; the key is to pack the bomb tightly. Let the bombs dry overnight.

Store in an airtight container away from heat and sunlight. To use, just place one on the floor of your shower.

DOUGLAS FIR PESTO

I love pesto so much I sometimes just eat a tiny scoop right off the spoon. The green, garlicky flavor lights up my insides and makes me do the happy food dance. My first pesto experiment was with stinging nettle leaves, and it turned out so good I just started to try random other plants that I thought might be tasty. This led me to Douglas fir pesto, a true wild forager's delight.

Items needed:
Food processor

Ingredients:
½ cup fresh spring Douglas fir tips
5 to 6 cloves of garlic, depending on size
¼ cup + 1 tbsp. pine nuts, gently roasted
¾ cup of olive oil
¼ cup minced Italian parsley
½ tsp. cumin
Lemon juice, to taste
Salt and pepper, to taste

Add all ingredients into the food processor and give it a few pulses to blend everything together. Then, with the food processor on low, slowly begin to add the olive oil. Pause to scrape down the sides of the bowl as necessary. Pulse just until blended. Adjust seasoning as desired.

Elder

Sambucus nigra

Family: Adoxaceae
Parts used: fruit,
leaf, bark
Medicinal actions:
Bark: diuretic, emet-
ic, purgative. *Leaves:*
diuretic. *Flowers:* dia-
phoretic. *Fruit:* antiviral,
aperient, immune
stimulation, tonic
Native geography:
Europe as far south
as Turkey, some parts
of Asia. Present in the
US except in Nevada,
Utah, Idaho, Oregon,
Washington, Alaska, and
Hawaii. Canada from
Manitoba east through
New Brunswick, Prince
Edward Island, and
Nova Scotia

I remember the first time I went to wild-craft elderberries. I had been working in my first herb shop, Wonderland Tea and Spice, for a while, and finally built up the courage to try foraging myself. As a newbie, it can be extremely intimidating to head out into the woods in search of a particular plant. Sure, I felt confident in the morning with my guidebook and map in hand, but when I finally parked the car and headed into the woods, doubt inevitably began to creep in. An acquaintance had shared a location where she'd previously harvested elderberries, so I was 90 percent sure I was in the right place. But that 10 percent of uncertainty kept my mind asking, "Are you sure you know what you are doing?" It reminded me of the time before cell phones, when driving directions would say "go about three miles." So you'd go what you thought were three miles, but start to think you must have overshot the next landmark, so you do a U-turn. You drive all the way back to where you started and do another U-turn only to drive thirty feet farther than you did for the first three miles and find where you actually needed to turn. That was a bit how I was feeling this first time wildcraft-ing for elderberries—looking for a specific tree in the woods felt equally vague.

It was October and one of those days where the clouds dominated most of the day, casting the forest in deep shades of green. When the sun came out for just a few moments, I'd stopped and turned my face upward to feel the last of its warmth. Somehow, that pause and dose of sun stopped time just long enough to let my intention for the day

come back. I reviewed what I was looking for: a tall, shaggy-looking shrub with compound, pinnate leaves. I read and reread the descrip-tion a dozen times in my field guide. I knew the leaves were pointed and sharply toothed. Elder is very easy to identify in the spring by its white showy display of flowers, but in fall it doesn't stand out in the same way.

As I continued searching, I spotted a few other herbal allies and decided to add them to my basket. That way if I came up empty-handed on the elder, at least I'd return with some hawthorn berries and rose hips for my ever-growing home medicine cabinet. Both those were easy to spot in the woods—their deep-red, tempting fruit popped out against the quickly turning browns and grays of the other vegetation.

I kept walking. Foraging is rarely accom-plished on an established trail. You must often go off the path to find the treasures of an herbal bounty. As a woman in her middle twenties, I couldn't help but feel that my searching in the woods was a bit of a metaphor for my life. The inner me was a wild bram-ble of flowers and thorns that I had to tease apart to make progress toward where I was going and what I was hoping to achieve. I was someone who often jumped off cliffs while naively assuming I'd always land safely on soft earth. I considered boundaries helpful, but felt that stepping outside of them had also led me to some of the most exquisite rewards. So as I stepped off the marked trail in search of elderberries, I felt hopeful. But here is where the fusion of planned execution of my task and reckless abandon met. Through the trials

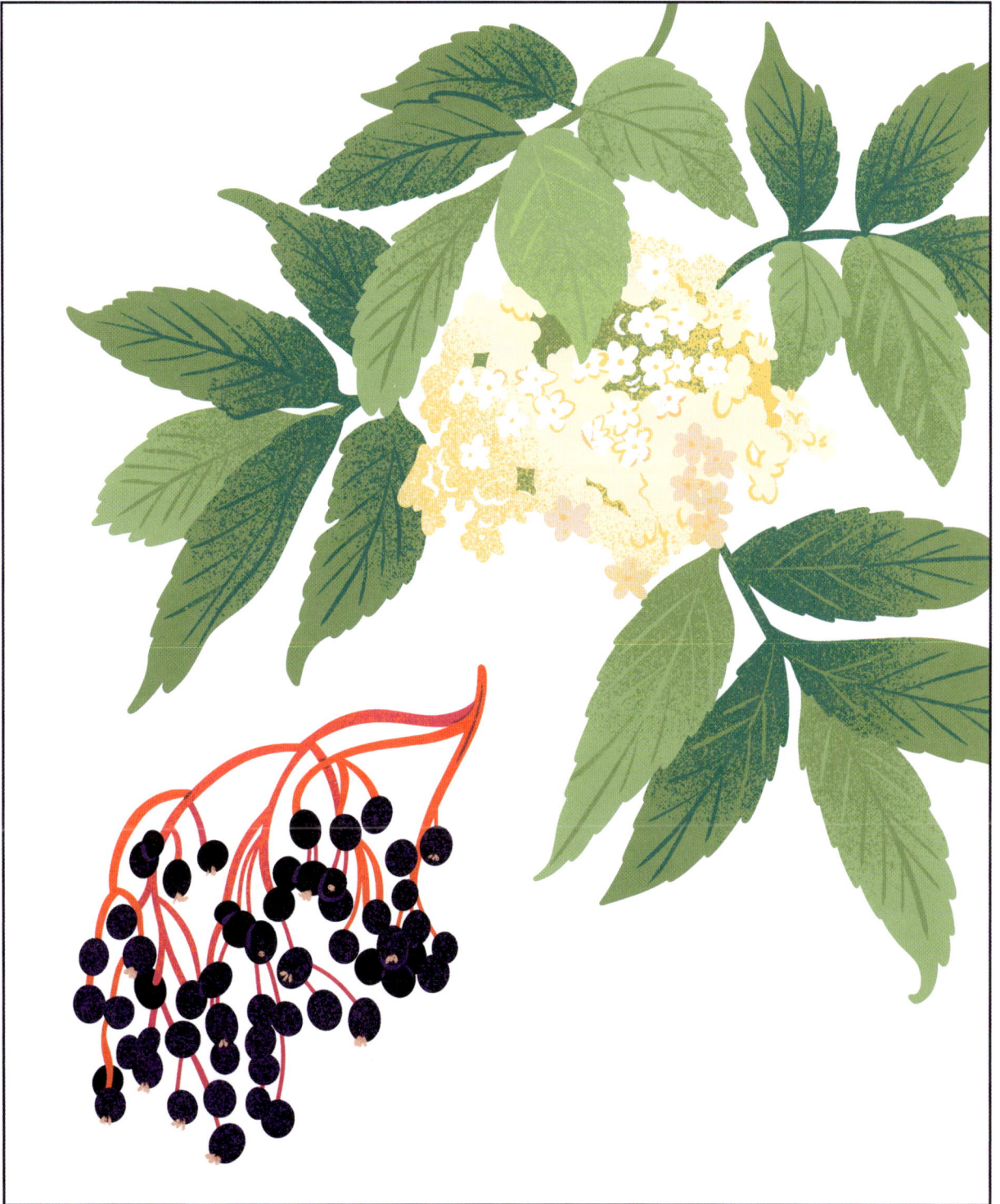

USDA hardiness
zones: 4 to 10
Water: keep soil consistently moist to wet
Light requirement: sun to part shade
Soil: tolerant of many soils, prefers moist humus
Temperature: able to survive to -20˚F
Wildlife notes: 48 species of birds eat the fruit, as do dormice and bank voles; moth caterpillars feed on elder foliage
Pollinator friendly: pollinated mainly by flies
Pests: canker, powdery mildew, leaf spot, borer

and errors involved in learning to wildcraft, I adopted defined techniques, practices, and consistency. Because using these skills usually resulted in success, I began to apply a similar discipline to other areas of my life and suddenly found purpose and direction.

Back in the woods, I could tell I was honing in on where I needed to be. My friend had warned me about an elder look-alike, pokeweed, in the same area, so when I saw that, I knew I was close. And then, there it was. I could see reddish stems set off by abundant blue berries from afar. As I got closer, I noticed the white powdery covering on the berries: it was a *Sambucus cerulea*, or blue elder. It was a large and beautiful tree, loaded and dripping with berries. I felt a bit surprised that I'd actually accomplished this quest. I felt a sense of pride, but at the same time the journey had been humbling. Ultimately, I felt gratitude. Through all the zigzags it had taken to get there, the universe had ultimately led me to this exact spot.

I quickly got to work harvesting, as it had taken the better part of the morning to find the elder. As I clipped the twigs and berry bunches, I let them fall gently into my collection basket. Simple pleasures make life rich. And a basket full of foraged elderberries is certainly a pleasure.

I've always used elder in the wintertime. I was taught that all its parts offer aid for the ailments of winter: colds, digestive complaints, fevers, and nerve pain. Harvesting the flowers in the early summer and berries in the fall is one forage I never want to miss. I've been making my annual elderberry syrup for over thirty years, and everyone in the family knows to reach for it as needed. The aroma that fills the home while I'm cooking elderberries is sweet

and reminiscent of my grandma. When my kids were young, I added a splash of elderberry syrup to their water bottles to fuel their bodies with extra flavonoids during the cold season.

In my thirties, I started to notice elderberry products popping up on the shelves at my grocery store, the nearby co-op, and drugstore. My first thought was, "Yay!" The population at large was finally ready to embrace another herb besides echinacea. But as with many things, poorly disseminated information in the form of commercial marketing has left the majority misled on how and when to use elderberry.

The elderberry plant has been considered a valuable medicine since the ninth century. Charlemagne, ruler and Christian Emperor of the West, decreed that an elder plant should be planted at every home. Perhaps it had aided him in a time of need or he bore witness to its medicinal effects; either way, elder became a household staple. Events such as this firmly root some herbs' reputation, and the legacy lasts centuries. Elders have consistently remained in favor for more than 1,200 years now—a great example of how herbal knowledge has been shared through generations.

We use the berry, bark, and the flowers as medicine. Traditionally, the berry was used for nerve discomforts such as back pain, sciatica, and neuralgia. It was also given to children in the form of a jam when lower digestive issues arose. Today we mostly see it as a syrup or capsules to be used to boost the immune system and fight colds and flu. Modern research has established that elder has a high bioflavonoid profile and an ability to inhibit certain viral strains, so it's now sold for that target market.

It may be worth planting your own home elder. Several cultivars of *Sambucus nigra* are widely available, all of which have a medicinal value. Each individual flower has 5 delicate petals that are creamy white and produce a musky scent. It is best to prune dead stems in the late winter. Plant may need to be 1 to 2 years old before berries emerge. *Sambucus nigra* are monoecious so are able to self-pollinate, but it has been found that having different varieties planted close by increases bloom and fruit. The flowers are a diaphoretic and a good choice when fever is present. They open up the pores to gently allow the fever to do its job, but comfort the patient by promoting sweating. The flower also has been shown to increase phagocytosis, the killing of foreign microorganisms in the body. I also add elderflower to certain circulation formulas as it seems to open up smaller vessels and improve microcirculation. The bark is only to be used in small doses, as it is a strong purgative and diuretic, but there are times when this might be desired. The leaves are also brewed to increase urination, or act like a diuretic when excess water of the body needs to be released.

Elder Recipes

INDICATIONS

- Bronchitis
- Circulation
- Colds
- Digestive
- Edema
- Fevers
- Flu
- Inflammation
- Nerve pain
- Pleurisy
- Sinusitis
- Viral infections

Generally regarded as safe for all populations. DO NOT consume raw berries, they need to be cooked or macerated to eliminate trace sambunigrin, a poisonous cyanogenic glycoside. Bark is only brewed fresh and should not exceed doses of 2 oz.

ELDERBERRY SYRUP

Very few herbs have as long of a written history as elderberry. These eye-catching berries must have caught the attention of herbal healers many centuries ago. Even Hippocrates, known as the Greek father of medicine, considered the elder tree a treasure. Herbalists have collected the berry to incorporate into various concoctions as well as delectable food creations. Throughout Europe you can still find elderberry pies for sale in local bakeries, and we know many tribes of Indigenous peoples used them for various ailments. I consider making elderberry syrup a herbalist initiation of sorts.

Items needed:
Stockpot
Large glass measuring cup
Strainer
Muslin cloth
Glass storage bottles

Ingredients:
4 cups fresh elderberries
8 cups water
Honey or organic cane sugar
Apple cider vinegar (optional)

Put the elderberries in the stockpot and bring it to a boil. Stir, then turn the heat to medium-low. Partially cover the pot with a lid, ensuring that it is ajar to allow for evaporation. At this point, stir every few minutes and simmer until you have reduced the overall volume in the pot by half. Let cool slightly.

Place the strainer over the large glass measuring up and strain the berry decoction. Compost the discarded berries or better yet, give them to your chickens if you have them. Line the strainer with a muslin cloth and strain the liquid a second time. Measure the volume of liquid that has been collected.

Next, return the decoction to a freshly cleaned stockpot and add honey or cane sugar in a 1:1 ratio of elderberry decoction to sweetener. So if you have 2 cups of decoction, then you'd add 2 cups of sugar. Gently heat, stirring constantly until all sugar is dissolved. Be sure to not overheat or scald the liquid, especially if you are using honey, as this could kill the active enzymes. If you'd like to add apple cider vinegar, now is the time. Add a 1:4 ratio of decoction to apple cider vinegar and stir. Allow the syrup to cool, then bottle and store in a cool, dark place or the refrigerator. Shelf life is typically 2 to 3 months.

ELDERBERRY SAUCE

Do you have a favorite cake or scone recipe that needs a special spread? Or how about a yummy vanilla ice cream topper? Here is the perfect thing.

Items needed:
Ceramic saucepan
Immersion blender
1 16-oz. glass jar, or 2 8-oz. jars

Ingredients:
2 cups fresh elderberries
2 tbsp. freshly squeezed lemon juice
½ cup packed organic brown sugar
½ cup organic cane sugar
1 to 2 tsp. vanilla extract
¼ tsp salt
¼ tsp cinnamon

Begin by simmering the berries and lemon juice, covered, on low. Check every couple of minutes and stir to ensure they aren't getting browned on the bottom.

Next, stir in the sugars, extract, salt, and cinnamon and simmer for another few minutes to blend flavors and slightly thicken. Stir often and ensure heat is low but sauce is simmering. Turn off the heat and let it cool slightly.

With an immersion blender, give the mixture just a few zips. The idea is to have a slightly smooth consistency but with some lumps and bumps for texture. Scoop into jars, label, and store in the refrigerator.

Elm

Ulmus americana

Family: Ulmaceae
Parts used: phloem
(the inner bark)
Medicinal actions:
demulcent, diuretic,
emollient, nervine, tonic
Native geography:
concentrated in North
Carolina in North Amer-
ica, but can be found
from southwestern
Maine west to New York,
northern Michigan, cen-
tral Minnesota, and east-
ern North Dakota, south
to eastern South Dakota,
central Nebraska, south-
western Oklahoma, and
central Texas, then east
to northwestern Florida
and Georgia

When I was thirteen my dad, an econo-
mist, suddenly decided he wanted to
be a farmer. He announced this at one
of our awkward Tuesday night dinners. My
mom and dad had divorced three years earlier,
but they decided to have weekly dinners with
the new blended families. These included dad,
his new wife, her two teenage sons, and me. As
a teen, I always found them uncomfortable, to
say the least. It followed that Tuesday nights
were also when "family" decisions would be
shared. He told us he had already bought a
farm outside of town and was moving in a
month. I envisioned horses and cute farm animals, like pigs and chickens. I couldn't wait to
see what kind of barn was on the property and
instantly started a list in my head of all the
cute farm activities we'd do. A few weeks later,
we all loaded up in the car and drove thirty
minutes south. As we drove through the town
of Bennet, Nebraska, all I saw was a feed store,
a few abandoned buildings, and a railroad
crossing. Where were the quilt shop and the
quaint general store? Where was the little café
where farmers gathered around to drink their
coffee and shoot the shit? Bennet was not the
idyllic country town I'd imagined, but I was
still sure the new farm would be charming.

I could barely contain my excitement as
my dad drove over a drainage ditch onto our
new driveway. We hadn't talked much along
the way, my dad's preference while driving, so
we did what we always did: listened to classical
music. The only genre my dad ever listened to.
When I got out of the car, I did not see a barn,
or corrals, or green pastures. All I saw were
huge swaths of overgrown shrubs and grass. It

looked like a wild field littered with abandoned junk. Where was the white picket fence,
the rolling hills? A tan house squatted on the
property; it was neither pretty nor inviting.
All I could think was, "But where am I going
to put my horse?"

My dad brought out the Braunschweiger
sandwiches he'd packed to "surprise" us for a
picnic. Since he hadn't brought a blanket or
chairs, though, we sat on the warm pavement
of the driveway. It was here he laid out his
plan. First, we'd all work the entire summer to
clear the land. *Ummmm, excuse me?* We'd have
to dig up all the grass and weeds and create
pathways to the gardens he had planned. We'd
mow, we'd rototill, we'd hoe fields and build
pergolas. I wondered where I could look up
laws about child labor.

I wound up being assigned to mow,
which was fun at first, because I used a riding
mower and so I got to learn to "drive," but for
a teenager, the chore quickly grew tiresome. I
learned how to use a rototiller, too. I only got
sunstroke once. My dad's wife had collected
thousands of heavy and thick concrete pavers,
and she waved her hands around as we walked,
showing us where she wanted pathways. "No
problem," I thought. "I can just lay them where
she wants them to go, and over time, with us
walking repeatedly on them, they'll sink into
place." I was quickly corrected and shown how
we needed to dig perfect rectangles for each
in the earth below, for stability. At this point,
I began to wonder when my allowance was
going to increase.

Then came building a vegetable cellar.
On one side of a berm to the north of the

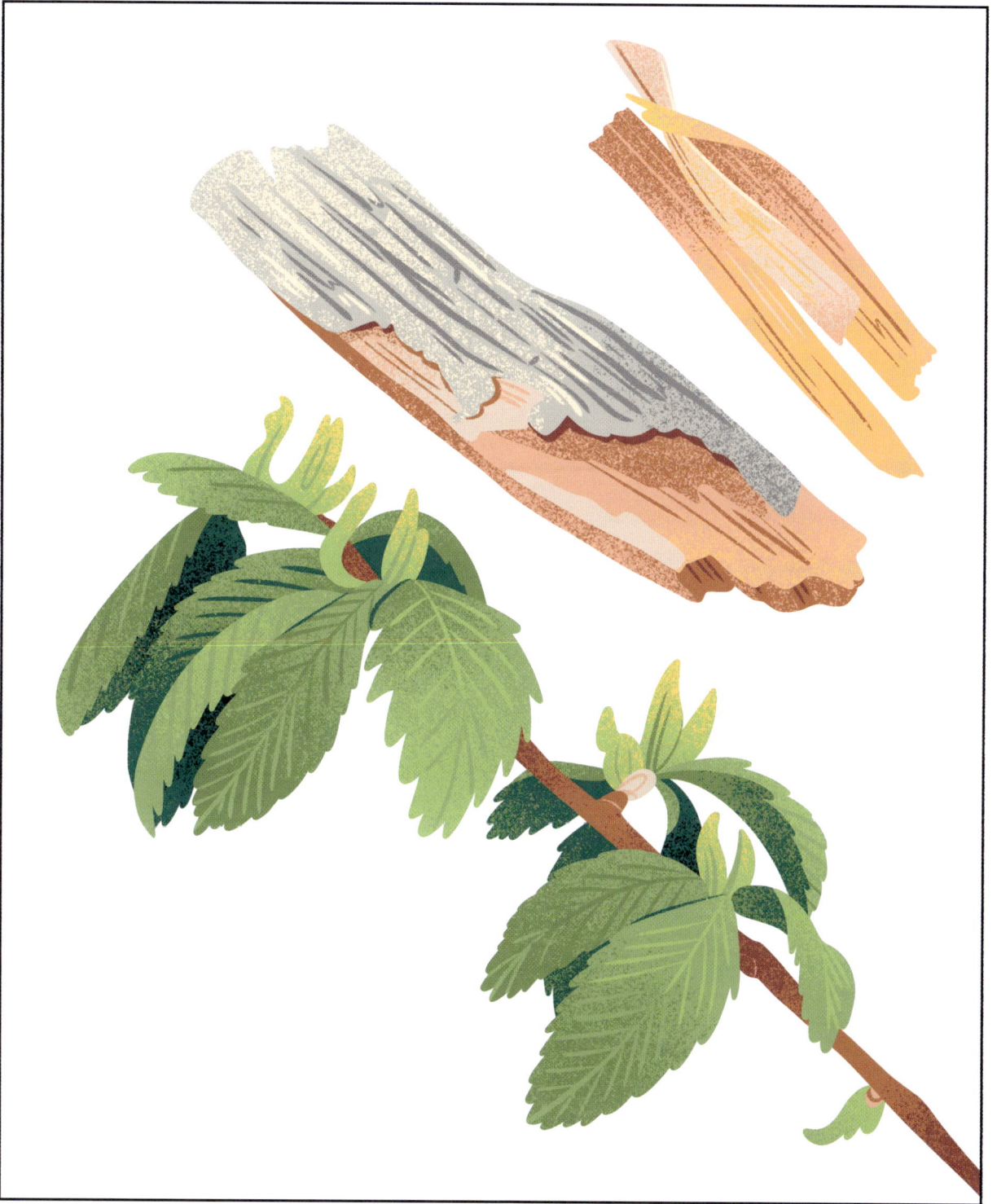

**USDA hardiness
zones:** 3 to 7
Water: water sparingly
Light requirement:
sun to part shade
Soil: Prefers well-
drained soil but can be
grown in sandy, loamy,
or even clay soils
Temperature: Hardy
to -35°F
Wildlife notes: a food
source for the ques-
tion mark butterfly; is
a larvae host for the
mourning cloak moth
and Columbia silkmoth
Pollinator friendly:
pollinated by wind
Pests: susceptible to
Dutch elm disease
and elm yellows

house there was an old creepy hole—someone had previously had the same idea, but never finished the project. It had loads of cobwebs, which meant there were spiders I couldn't see. It smelled of damp earth, but not in the pleasant "petrichor" way—more like in the rotting abyss way. But my dad had long since closed the complaints department. We were each handed a shovel. I essentially spent my weekend visits digging dirt.

During that first visit to "the farm," after I realized there was no barn and ergo no future horse, I set my sights on the one thing that felt familiar: a tree. A big, beautiful American elm tree grew over what someday would be our flower garden. I'd always been a tree climber, finding peace and solitude among the branches. There is no better place to get perspective than from sitting up in a tree. This elm was tall, so I had to use a white plastic lawn chair to reach its lowest branch. I wrapped my arms around it, pretending I was on the monkey bars, then hoisted myself up and ascended three or four more branches. (I'd kill to be able to do that now, at my age.) I looked out over the land, and I could see that the neighbors down south had hundreds of beehives. I could see the tiny creek that bordered our property to the west. And I actually spotted a gray speckled horse up on the horizon to the north. To the east was the road that took me back to my mom's. I could see my second family milling around below me, looking this way and that, considering my dad's master plan. From up here I could almost believe in it and picture it, finished.

———

Ulmus rubra, otherwise known as slippery elm, is a tried-and-true friend in the medicine cabinet. It's safe enough for the entire family, from young to old. Slippery elm is the inner

bark, often taken from smaller branches and fallen trees. It's an excellent choice any time you need to calm irritated mucous mem-branes. Think sore throats, heartburn, IBS, or Crohn's disease, just to name a few. Areas of the body along the digestive tract produce mucous when they are out of balance or inflamed. The natural production of mucous in these areas is meant to be protective, to soothe irritation caused by a virus, bacteria, food sensitivity, or allergy.

When acute illness occurs, as in the case of strep throat, the invading bacteria multiplies quickly. So quickly that the body doesn't have the means to eradicate it before it settles in. Other times, when chronic or recurring illness is present, such as with IBS, the intestines are in a constant state of inflammation, and the protective mucous production gradually declines.

In any of these situations, slippery elm is extremely helpful. It acts as a demulcent, an emollient, and a nutritive all at the same time. Herbs that provide relief from inflammation while at the same time offering nutritive benefits are definitely those you should keep on hand. A lot of the time we are targeting symptoms when we get sick. I have a headache = I want the pain in my head to go away. Or, I have a cold = get rid of my runny nose. But if you add in tonic or nutritive herbs for the headache or runny nose, while at the same time treating the symptom, you are making the affected systems stronger.

With slippery elm you not only have a symptom reliever, but a tonic as well. When we use it for digestive issues, it can alleviate pain by soothing the tissues, coating the area to ensure the inflammation isn't damaging the tissues, and nourishing the tissues with nutrients. I use slippery elm all the time. I add it to congee or porridge as a nutritive boost for those convalescing. I apply it topically mixed with plantain for any type of skin issue: wound, abscess, boil. And, blended with a touch of licorice root, it makes my kids' favorite tea. Slippery elm has calcium, which contributes to alleviating the previously mentioned complaints. But it also has been used in supporting emotional well-being. Those with a manic-depressive tendency have also benefited from it.

American elm and slippery elm look very similar; the best way to tell them apart is to look at the leaves. American elm leaves come to a rounded point, whereas the slippery elm leaf has a small, extended, pointed leaf at the end. Some have compared it to a little tail. It's best to harvest slippery elm in the spring, when the sap flow has begun. The outer bark will typically slip right off then, and the phloem will have a higher concentration of minerals and nutrients. Then you need to separate the outer bark from the inner bark. The outer bark is soft, whereas the inner bark is fibrous. Dry the inner bark for later use. If possible, harvest only from fallen trees or broken branches as the phloem forms part of the tree's active "circulatory" system, moving sugars produced in the leaves during photosynthesis to other parts of the tree used for growth or for storage, so cutting it away can damage a living tree.

Elm Recipes

INDICATIONS

- Bronchitis
- Constipation
- Cough
- Crohn's disease
- Diarrhea
- Diverticulitis
- Dyspepsia
- Heartburn
- Hemorrhoids
- IBS
- Mood swings
- Skin: abscess, boil, wounds
- Sore throat
- Stomach ulcers

*Ulmus rubra is declining in the wild. Please be responsible if wildcrafting and harvest only from fallen trees or downed branches. Use for a period of 2-3 weeks if using for a chronic condition, then stop to evaluate effectiveness.

SLIPPERY ELM JUICE

When I first started practicing herbalism, I was twenty-two years old. I didn't need slippery elm for digestive complaints and lumped it, along with a few other herbs into the "old person" category. Well here I am, thirty years later, lapping up the "old person juice."

This is a tried-and-true recipe for anyone suffering from almost any type of digestive issue. Chronic inflammation of the GI tract is soothed by the slippery elm and can help to heal the mucosal lining. If you are fighting a digestive bacterial infection, consider adding the optional goldenseal and licorice.

Items needed:
Saucepan
Strainer
Glass measuring cup

Ingredients:
2 tbsp. slippery elm bark
1 tbsp. comfrey root
½ tsp. cinnamon bark
1-2 tbsp. honey or maple syrup to sweeten
Optional ½ tsp. goldenseal powder, ¼ tsp. licorice root powder

Bring 2 cups of water to a boil, then add slippery elm and comfrey root. Reduce heat and simmer, covered, for 5 minutes. Turn off the heat and add optional goldenseal and licorice root if desired. Give a stir, cover, and let steep for 15 minutes.

Strain and return to the saucepan. Add sweetener if you'd like. The consistency should be a bit thick. Store in a glass bottle in the refrigerator for up to 4 days. Drink 1- to 2-tablespoon doses three to four times a day.

SLIPPERY ELM GUT HEALTH SMOOTHIE

This smoothie promotes gentle digestion by soothing the tummy and calming the gastrointestinal tract. Slippery elm is a nutritive natural emollient, supporting proper health all along the digestive tract.

Items needed:
Blender

Ingredients:
½ cup of yogurt, dairy or nondairy
½ banana
2 tbsp. pineapple juice or ¼ cup of diced pineapple
¼ aloe vera juice
1 tbsp. slippery elm powder
½ tbsp. psyllium husk powder
¼ cup water or milk of choice
3 or 4 ice cubes

Blend all ingredients together in the blender until smooth. Enjoy.

SLIPPERY ELM LATTE

When you aren't feeling your best and the throat is feeling sore, why not skip the coffee and help the body out? Try this latte to soothe the throat fire.

Items needed:
Saucepan
Bowl
Whisk
Immersion blender, if you have one

Ingredients:
1 tbsp. slippery elm bark powder
½ cup milk, dairy or nondairy
1 cup water
1 tbsp. maple syrup or honey
¼ cinnamon powder
¼ cardamom powder
⅛ clove powder
Sprinkle of nutmeg

Bring ½ cup of milk to a simmer and pour into a ceramic bowl. Add 1 cup of water to the pan and bring to a boil.

In the meantime, add the slippery elm to the milk slowly and whisk to blend. You can also use a few zaps of a drink mixer but either way, don't over mix.

Once the water is boiling, turn off the heat and add the milk/slippery elm blend to the water. Once again, give a quick whisk. Add the sweetener and spices and whisk again. Pour into a mug and sprinkle with nutmeg.

Note: you can also add the slippery elm to the water and froth the milk if you prefer.

Eucalyptus

Eucalyptus globulus

Family: Myrtaceae
Parts used: leaves
Medicinal actions:
antibacterial, antiviral, antiseptic, decongestant, deodorant, expectorant, febrifuge, stimulant
Native geography:
southeastern Australia; the species was introduced into California in 1856 and Hawaii around 1865 and has become naturalized in both states; it also grows well in the southern regions of Spain, Portugal, and Peru

Ollantaytambo sits at 2,792 feet above sea level in the Cusco region of the sacred valley in Peru. It is a warm, welcoming town, rich in cultural history. I fell in love with it the first time I visited. I had been making my way to Aguas Calientes, the entry point to Machu Picchu, and stayed with a friend next to the train station.

I've always loved places that have town squares. They create easy landmarks for meeting points and seem to function as a true heart of the town. In Ollantaytambo, many shops line the edges of the square, with plenty of places to sit in either the sun or shade to relax and say hello to passersby. Musicians sometimes play, and kids constantly run around, often kicking a ball between them. As a traveler, I find town squares the best place to sit, enjoy a tea, and write. Even with the periodic distractions, witnessing everyday life reminds us that we are actually living, and not just moving along in the construct of a life.

I'd heard of a hike outside of town that started at an archaeological site considered to be older than Machu Picchu. Pumamarca was once a fortress said to have been the gateway into the Sacred Valley. For five US dollars, a taxi would drive me up to the site, and then I could take my time walking down the trail back to town. I packed up my water bottle, a snack, my camera, and notebook. After a relatively quick drive, passing farms and driving up gravel roads, I was let out among crumbling structures and ancient rock buildings.

I spent the better part of two hours walking around. I like to feel spaces out. I like to touch the rock walls and sit in old rooms to journal. Pumamarca sits higher than Ollantaytambo, at 11,000 feet; you feel perceptibly closer to the sky. A flat plateau overlooks the valley below, and the view from there is transcendental. I focused on breathing in and out in the thin air while my eyes scanned the terrain taking in green mountains, rivers, cattle, llamas, dogs, people, laundry drying, crops…so much life.

But as with any hike, there comes a time to head back. It was difficult to leave, knowing that once I descended, I'd return to normalcy, losing the view and the feeling. With reluctance, I chose what I thought was the path. Here there are no neatly marked trails. Worn footpaths cut through pastures, past bulls who lazily look up as you move by, over creeks with banks full of unexpected flowers, trees, and plants. As I made my way, I kept seeing the most beautiful blue-green seed pods under my feet. I recognized them as belonging to the eucalyptus, or blue gum tree, and then noticed they were growing all around me. My first thought was confusion, because I know they are not native to Peru. But there they were, their aroma filling the air; they waved their sickle-shaped leaves at me as I passed by.

Suddenly, I remembered a poem by Robinson Jeffers. A prolific poet and environmentalist, he once penned fourteen beautiful lines giving gratitude for the eucalyptus tree. In one of the verses he recognizes the journey this global tree has taken, having made its way from Australia to far lands. I wondered whether these very eucalyptus trees had also been brought over as saplings, as offerings or gifts? Or had they actually originated here and

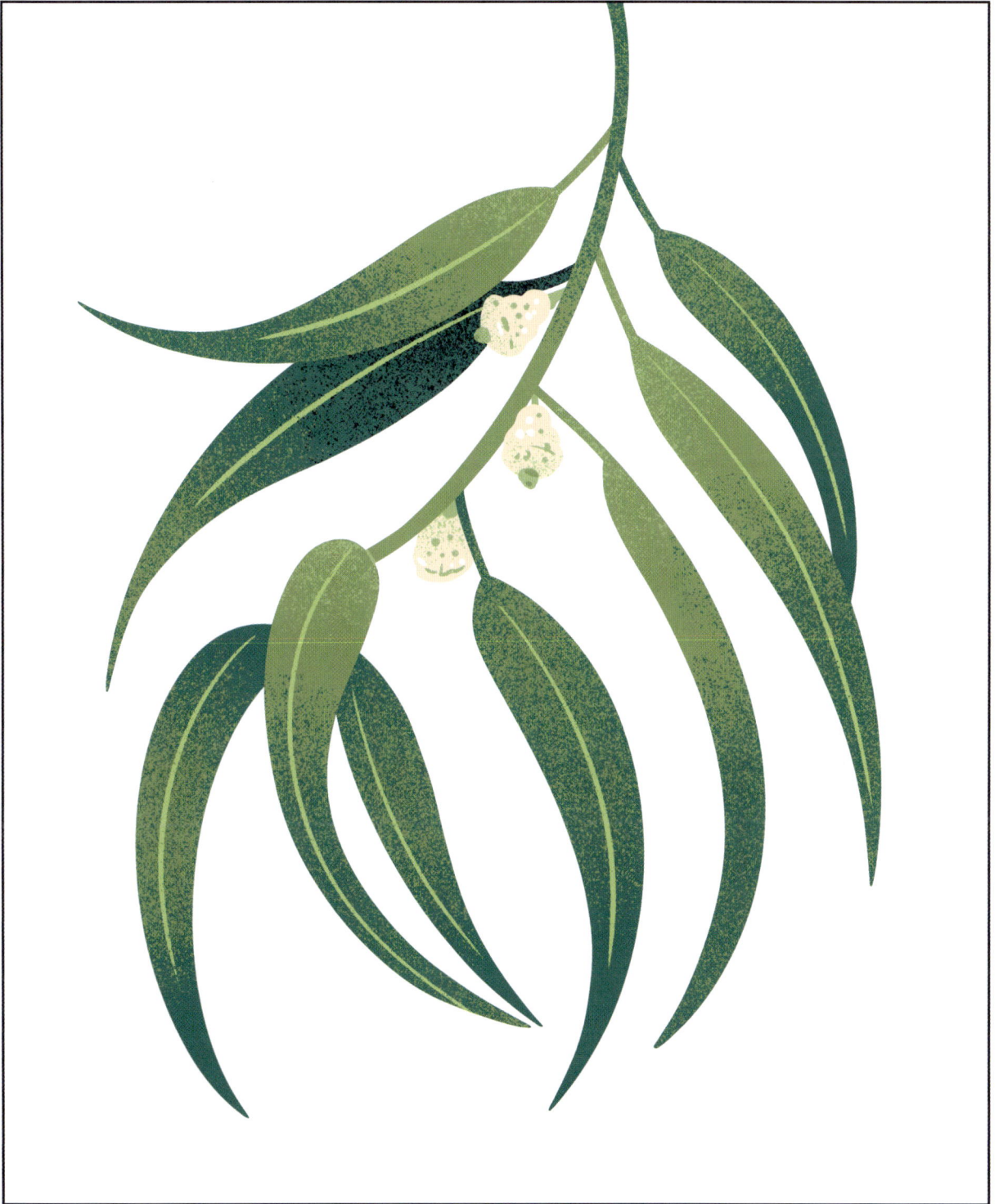

**USDA hardiness
zones:** 8 to 11b
Water: happiest in
moist soil but can
tolerate drought
Light requirement:
full sun
Soil: good drainage, low
salinity, and a topsoil
depth of 2 feet or more
Temperature: frost
resistance increases
with maturity
Wildlife notes: Koalas
eat eucalyptus leaves
Pollinator friendly:
in zones where eucalyp-
tus blooms year round, it
attracts bees and gives
their honey a distinctive
peppermint-like taste
Pests: beetles, psyllids,
and beetle borers

made their way to Australia? I kept wondering about the intricate and strong seeds as I
walked. Much like precious acorns, I couldn't
resist picking up a few (or fifty). They are
the most curious-looking things: a dimpled
blue-white cone sits on top of a round, brown,
button-like seed with four slits that make me
think of the top of a pie. I kept envisioning
them being used as the heads and hats of
tiny nature dolls that my Waldorf-school
kids might craft. When I reached the home
again and opened my bag, the smell greeted
me. I was instantly transported back to Peru.
My mind, body, and soul were grasping to
re-create the feeling I had looking out from
Pumamarca.

———————

Eucalyptus trees provide scent throughout
the year, wherever they grow. It's a deciduous
tree that sheds its bark annually. My favorite
part of the tree is the fruit—they are cone-
shaped and rough on the outside. Some refer
to them as "warty," but to me that doesn't
quite fit. When fresh they are blue, but later
turn brown.

Eucalyptus leaves are a powerful antiseptic and astringent. They clear away gunk and
pull tissues together. Because of the powerful
constituent eucalyptol, modern medicine
strongly advises not to consume eucalyptus.
But in traditional herbalism, including
small amounts in tea formulas was common.
Eucalyptus alleviates head and respiratory
congestion and can be a lifesaver for sinusitis.
The confusion may lie with the popularity of
eucalyptus essential oil, which is toxic when
consumed. Essential oils are very concentrated; this has eucalyptol and hydrocyanic
acid. Also, eucalyptus oil is rapidly absorbed
into the bloodstream, so toxicity symptoms as
severe as coma and death can arise quickly.

The leaves, however, have many beneficial
applications. Making an herbal inhalation
steam with eucalyptus leaves opens up the
nasal passageways and relieves congestion
pressure. Add some rosemary and thyme
along with it and you've got a super-packed
antiviral, antibacterial vapor that will attack
almost anything in the respiratory tract. I
often put some in a muslin bag, tie it around
the spigot, and make a bath for my kids with
it when they have a cold. The hot water from
the bath creates a medicinal steam and as they
splash around, it stimulates the release of the
oil from the leaves.

Making an herbal oil with the leaves
will produce a great addition to any type of
homemade vapor balm. I grew up with Vicks
VaporRub™ as a kid; the idea is similar, but as
a mom and adult decided the petroleum base
wasn't for me. I now make a beeswax-based
vapor rub with eucalyptus oil as a main
ingredient. Herbal oil is different from
essential oil; it's created by slow-cooking the
leaves in olive oil for four to six hours over a
very low flame. An essential oil is created by
heating the leaves in a distiller and collecting
the oil from the vapor, which results in a
much more concentrated solution. I typically
rub my vapor rub on the chest and top of the
back (where the top of the lungs are) before
bed. Sometimes I'll lay a hot towel over that
area to increase the vapor release. Eucalyptus
leaves relax the respiratory tract to aid in the
expulsion of phlegm and mucous.

Eucalyptus leaves are strongly scented,
so if they're used in quantity in any tea blend,
they can easily overtake the flavor profile.
I recommend including leaves as no more
than 10 percent of your total blend of tea
ingredients. A simple example of a cold tea
would be a mix of 40 percent elderflower, 40
percent peppermint, 10 percent hyssop, and
10 percent eucalyptus.

The essential oil is very useful too. If you happen to have an essential oil distiller around, I definitely recommend utilizing it with your harvest of eucalyptus leaves. I often put a little on my kids' feet before bed when they have a cold or add a few drops to a diffuser in their room. It is also known to aid in wound healing, for relieving aches and joint pain, balancing blood sugar, and soothing cold sores.

Eucalyptus Recipes

INDICATIONS

- Abscesses
- Balances blood sugar
- Bronchitis
- Circulation
- Colds
- Cold sores
- Congestion
- Coughs, especially spasmodic cough
- Fever
- Flu
- Joint pain
- Sinusitis
- Wound healing

NOT FOR INTERNAL CONSUMPTION. *Essential oil is toxic and ingestion of large quantities of leaf as tea can cause toxicity. Add to a diffuser or blend with a bit of olive oil and apply topically. Asthmatics should use with caution.*

EUCALYPTUS BATH SALTS

When I have a head cold, nothing feels better than taking a hot bath with vibrant scents. The hot water warms my bones and the aromatic oils travel up to my sinuses to offer relief from congestion. Eucalyptus shines in this scenario, and when you blend it with a few other herbs you can create a luxury spa experience right in your own home.

Note: if you prefer a recipe where everything dissolves and drains from the tub, consider either grinding the eucalyptus leaves or use 40 or 50 drops of eucalyptus oil instead. Be sure to use a drain strainer if using crushed leaves.

Items needed:
Large mixing bowl
Mixing spoon
Storage containers

Ingredients:
4 cups epsom salt
1 cup Himalayan salt
1 cup Dead Sea salt
2 tbsp. baking soda
4 tbsp. dried, crushed eucalyptus leaves
4 tbsp. olive oil

Mix all ingredients in a large mixing bowl, tossing and stirring until everything is well combined. Put the mixture in a large quart-size mason jar with a small scoop to keep in the bathroom. You can also put it into smaller jars, cosmetic pouches, or even test tubes to give as gifts.

EUCALYPTUS TABLE GARLAND

I love a decorated dinner table. While I am no Martha Stewart, it is my belief that little touches make a table beautiful and a meal memorable. A garland of fresh eucalyptus instantly transforms a plain table. As the base you can use a few long craft sticks, but if you have a long twig or small branch from an alder, cedar, poplar, pine, or even grapevines, use that. Basically any branch that is as long as you want your garland to be will do. Add whatever colors you or coordinate with the seasons.

Items needed:
Base stick(s)
Floral wire
Wire cutters

Ingredients:
8 to 10 eucalyptus branches, 1 to 2 feet long (these are especially
    pretty if they have gone to seed as the seed umbels give the
    garland dimension and texture)
10 to 20 flowers of choice, such as baby's breath, tea roses, or mums
3 or 4 willow branches

Begin by laying the stick down on a large surface. Place the eucalyptus next to it, trying different arrangements until you find one you find attractive. Use wire cutters to precut the floral wire into two to three dozen pieces, each 3-4 inches long. Having them ready to go makes the next step easier.

First, mark your stick halfway down its length. Then slide the stick underneath your arranged eucalyptus and begin to wrap your wire around the eucalyptus to secure it to the stick. Overlap the branches slightly to cover up the wire and to give it some dimension. Once you reach the halfway mark of the stick, stop. Repeat from the opposite end. This creates a center focal point where the opposite ends meet in the middle.

Next, add additional types of flowers or vegetation if you wish. Use the floral wire to secure flowers or willow branches to increase the volume and texture of the garland.

Ficus

Ficus religiosa

Family: Moraceae
Parts used: bark,
fruit, leaves
Medicinal actions:
Bark and leaves: anti-
bacterial, antitussive,
astringent, hepatopro-
tective, immunostimu-
lant, vermifuge.
Fruit: laxative.
Native geography:
the Indian subcontinent
and Southeast Asia;
introduced but now
considered invasive
in Texas

I have a ficus tree growing in my bedroom. It started out as most of my houseplants do, a tiny little thing that I most likely found at a grocery store or some other random retailer. I had already killed one ficus; it started off happy and healthy and did well for a couple of years. But then I moved, and it endured two assaults. First, a friend who was helping me move put it in the back of his pickup truck and drove thirty minutes down a cold and windy highway. When I saw him pull up, I could immediately tell the plant was unhappy. Ficus are known to be temperamental; I could practically feel judgment oozing from this plant at that moment. I wondered if it would die just out of spite. The second assault was its new home. The light just wasn't the same as it had been. It was no longer in the same temperature environment or next to its other plant friends. I tried scooting it to different positions, but it finally gave up and died. You may think I didn't pick the right circumstance for it, but the more time I study plants, the more I believe that their emotional connection to us and their environment matters to their health.

When I was in my twenties, I had a small collection of ferns and philodendrons that filled the little nooks and crannies of my studio apartment. I lived in a studio in an old Victorian house. It had windows with lattice panes in the front, which I thought were so charming then. Now, in my fifties, I would immediately associate them with drafts. I set a lot of my plants on windowsills and ledges, surfaces that didn't have room for water trays. Live and learn.

Now it is time to disclose a personal secret, one that has frustrated many house-mates. No matter how hard I try to avoid it—and when I was younger I didn't try that hard—whenever I water houseplants, I always spill the water or overfill the pot. It's inevitable, even today. Because I had wall-to-wall carpet at the time, and that carpet was very, very old, I decided it was best for a new plan of action. I came up with the idea to gather all my plants and put them into the bathtub to have what I called a "houseplant party." I'd squeeze them all into my clawfoot tub, turn on whatever music fit the vibe, and start gently spraying them down with my handheld shower. I'd sing as I bathed them and ensured the water completely saturated the soil. Call me crazy, you won't be the first, but right from the get-go I noticed a difference. I'd swear they were vibrating and communicating in a way I could virtually feel. Plants that normally sat across the apartment from each other got to get up close and personal with each other. So began a weekly ritual. I even started rotating which plants I bathed together so they could all interact.

Research ficus, and you'll see that just about everyone says they are moody and overemotional. Yet sometimes, including in the wild, they grow freely and flourish. In *The Secret Life of Plants*, Peter Tompkins discusses the emotional terrain of plants. He cites solid research to justify the belief that plants do, in fact, have emotions. I think that some houseplants are

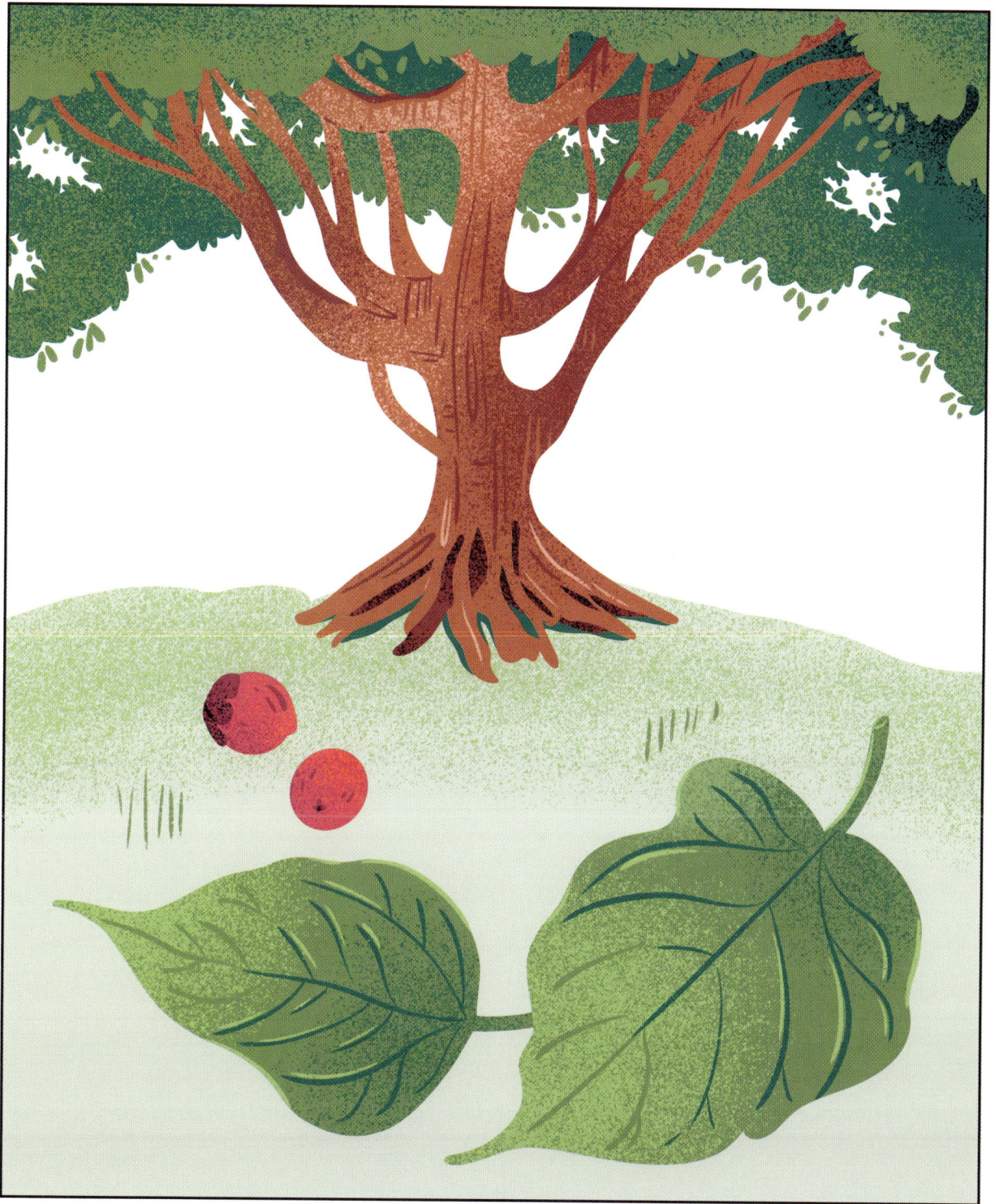

PLANT DATA
USDA hardiness zones: 10 to 12
Water: minimal watering; allow the soil to dry out between watering sessions
Light requirement: sun to part shade, or shade if in a subtropical zone
Soil: prefers well-drained soil, but can live in a variety of soil types
Temperature: intolerant of frost
Wildlife notes: birds, such as koels, sunbirds, and the kingfisher love this tree
Pollinator friendly: *Blastophaga quadriceps*, an agaonid wasp, is a coevolved pollinator for this species
Pests: fairly pest resistant

hard to grow because they are simply just sensitive, just like humans. Anyone who's tried to grow a fiddle-leaf fig or get an orchid to repeat bloom can relate. When you take a perfectly happy human and bring disruption or chaos into their lives, it can result in behavioral change. I think we are all (plant and human) born into a world as perfect as can be; it is our environment and level of care that determines whether we will survive, thrive, and develop.

One of my favorite aspects of traveling is to see plants growing wild in their native lands. Ficuses often act like an evergreen in tropical zones, never losing their leaves. They are fast-growing and, when mature, they become stately trees with a grand spread. Their heart-shaped, dark green glossy leaves identify them immediately. But what steals the show are the long aerial roots that descend from the canopy; when these eventually reach the ground, they act as mini-trunks, providing stability for the tree as it grows. The fruits and flowers grow directly out of the trunk or branches in a phenomenon known as "cauliflory" and bloom in shades of orange and red.

I am always in awe when I see specimens of the carefully tended houseplants I have at home living in the wild, thriving without any human intervention—I've seen some with trunks that were nearly ten feet wide. I often get introspective thinking about how well something grows when it is left to its own devices in an appropriate environment that naturally provides everything it needs. When we take a plant out of its preferred habitat, move it to a different climate, and expect it to perform for us, I can't help but feel we've lost a bit of our perception of reality. What if, just like our subtropical plants, all humans started out with just the right soil, water, compost, and sunlight to thrive?

My current (second) ficus has lived in the same pot, in the same spot, for ten years. Interestingly, it's placed next to a Boston fern that had nearly died three times before I moved to the farm and finally left it in one place. In 2010 it was down to one scraggly frond; I've since dedicated many hours to its revival. I swear the two plants are best friends. They sit quietly side by side, thriving and spilling water all over the floor.

Let's talk a little bit about meditation. After all, *Ficus religiosa* is said to be the tree the Buddha was sitting under when he achieved enlightenment. I'm always curious to see how people react to the idea of meditation. Does it make you roll your eyes and instantly turn you off? Does it make you think about all the times you've thought it would be a good practice to start, but you never manage? Or is meditation already a part of your regular routine?

There are many definitions of meditation. According to the Cleveland Clinic, meditation is a practice that involves focusing or clearing your mind using a combination of mental and physical techniques. Undoubtedly that's how some people practice. Personally, I meditate in many different ways, and most do not involve sitting in one place with my eyes closed. I find the easiest way to clear my mind in order to tap into my subconscious is simply to be out in nature. A walk in the forest close to my house takes my mind from churning to calm. The incessant messaging and racing thoughts that occur in the back of all our brains becomes more noticeable when other distractions are removed. It's like the stream I walk next to there, constantly flowing. I listen to this recorded replay for a while, taking notice of the key of my soundtrack. What I hear isn't always pleasant. Often, I just wish I could turn it off or at least turn it down. But that would defeat the purpose of the walk, right? So I stick with it. I sometimes bring a notebook and jot down what I'm feeling. I write things down when I hear my inner voice say something that surprises me, or when thoughts bring up emotions. For many, the simple act of putting feelings and thoughts down on paper frees up a lot of headspace.

When I feel calmer, like I've crossed through that barrier of brain chatter, I am able to look around and take in my environment. I notice the sounds of the birds, the creaking of the trees moving in the wind, the giant banana slugs that make their way across my path. I look at mushrooms and moss. I ponder how things have changed since the last time I was on the trail. All of this in an effort to get present. About three-quarters of the way through my usual loop, there is a bench. This is my meditating spot. I sit down . . . and do nothing. Whatever thoughts come, come. Whatever thoughts go, go. Maybe it is this practice, or this practice in combination with the ions and terpenes we breathe in in the forest (as an act of "forest bathing") that brings me to a point where I'm able to listen to my innermost voice. Not the monkey brain voice, but the one that resides deep inside of me.

For some, sitting still is an incredible entry to a meditative state. For others, exercise is a way to tap in. I often think about marathon runners and wonder if they are in deep meditation as they run for twenty-six miles. Or take Diana Nyad, who swam from Cuba to Florida. Was she in a steady state of meditation induced by the rhythm of her own strokes? The classic conception that meditation means sitting on a pillow with your eyes closed isn't for everyone. I think there is room to expand the way in which we practice, finding that quiet place in our own unique way.

Ficus Recipes

INDICATIONS

- Asthma
- Constipation
- Cough
- Diabetes
- Diarrhea
- Hemorrhage
- Liver tonic
- Parasites
- Skin complaints
- Ulcers
- Wound healing

*Generally regarded as safe for all populations.

FICUS RELIGIOSA RAITA

If you've never tried Indian raita, you are missing out. This cooling condiment has a many traditional variations—it can be made with dairy or without, for example, so feel free to substitute a plant-based yogurt. I don't recommend Greek yogurt, however, as it will create a sour taste. Eat it with roti bread or add it on top of virtually any dish. Feel free to play around with spices and proportions to accommodate your palate.

Items needed:
Saucepan
Strainer
Mixing bowl
Mixing spoon

Ingredients:
6 fresh ficus (pipal) leaves
1 cup plain yogurt
½ cup cucumber, diced
½ cup tomato, diced
¼ cup red onion, diced
½ tsp. organic unrefined sugar
½ tsp. coriander
½ tsp. cumin
¼ tsp. red pepper chili powder (optional)
Salt, to taste

First, add 4 cups of water to a saucepan and bring to a boil. Add the pipal leaves and turn off the heat. Stir until the leaves are soft, then strain. Dice the leaves and set aside.

Mix the yogurt, spices, and sugar together, then add the pipal leaves.

Add the cucumbers, tomato, and red onion and mix well. Chill for two hours before serving.

FICUS SKELETON LEAVES

Finding skeleton leaves in the forest always feels, to me, like a special gift—the exoskeleton of a leaf that is perfectly intact, leaving a geometric frame around where the green foliage used to be. This is also one of my kids' favorite decorative or seasonal projects.

There are several methods of making skeleton leaves; I prefer the old-fashioned way, which takes a bit of time. Sometimes having patience for 2 or 3 weeks is hard, especially when kids are involved, but I've found that they enjoy witnessing the transformation process.

Items needed:
Large bowl or dish; glass, plastic or ceramic
Shallow pan
Small paintbrush

Ingredients:
Ficus leaves

First, choose your leaves. For best results, select leaves that have a prominent, readily visible main vein. If the leaves are dirty, gently clean them in a bowl of warm water using a soft cloth or soft toothbrush.

Fill your baking dish or shallow pan with clean water and set it outside in the shade. You can also add soda bicarb, baking soda, bleach, or washing solution, but I find these to either be hard on the leaves or toxic to the environment. Next, add your leaves. It is okay if they overlap. Some may float to the top—just swish and rotate them daily. Every two or three days I gently lift the leaves out, dump the water, and refill the dish with clean water. After a week you can gently start to rub off decomposing plant material from the leaves as you are stirring. After two weeks, you can add a little water to the shallow pan and clean one leaf at a time with the small paintbrush.

Let the skeletons dry in the sun for two or three minutes before handling or using in a craft.

Ginkgo

Ginkgo biloba

Family: Ginkgoaceae
Parts used: leaves
Medicinal actions:
anti-inflammatory,
antioxidant, antitussive,
aphrodisiac, astringent,
cardioprotective, nerv-
ine, tonic, vasodilator,
vermifuge
Native geography:
China

I don't even remember why I had to go to the courthouse that day, but as I crossed Portland's park blocks, a dry rain of bright yellow leaves fell all around me. Once on the ground, they would get lifted by the wind again and sometimes create a deviling dervish I had to traverse to get to my destination. The brilliant color juxtaposed with the gray city buildings surrounding them made me pause, oscillate in my intention for the day. I had things to accomplish and an appointment to get to, but I would rather have sat in the park on a bench and taken in the autumn arriving before my very eyes.

There is something about fall that brings up deep emotions within me. Perhaps it is the residue of back-to-school memories. Or maybe it is the recollection of football games, the annual apple harvest, or even the lighting of the first fire in the fireplace. I'm sure it is this and 1,000 other moments in time that for one reason or another, mark the fall season as a particularly poignant one in my life. And although Nebraska, where I grew up, has an abundance of deciduous tree varieties, I don't recall any real memories of amazement regarding the changing of leaves in the fall there. Then again, I was young and the seasonal changes were probably about as high on my list of enthusiasms as birdwatching, which I thought was boring. It took until my thirties for me to even notice the changing of aspen leaves.

I'd never seen a ginkgo tree before moving to Portland. I'd used the leaves plenty in various herbal formulas, but had yet to see one alive and growing. That day, something took hold in me. A moment that required presence. I remember how all the urgency of my hustling and bustling fell away. There are more than two dozen ginkgo trees lining this particular street, creating a bright frame for the landscape all around it. They are all over fifty feet tall and stand close enough that their canopies touch, creating a continuous arch over the park, a living yellow tunnel. As I noticed the trunks of the trees, I recognized the deep dark browns of bark that only achieves such color if exposed to persistent dampness.

I had read that ginkgos are one of the oldest living tree species in the world and have existed practically unchanged for over 250 million years, so as I sat beneath one of the trees and looked up, I marveled that actual Jurassic-period dinosaurs had seen the same leaves. What makes this ancient species so resilient, while others have long since gone extinct? When I first went digging around for the answer to this question, I hypothesized theories such as adaptability and defense mechanisms against disease. Ginkgos are famous for having survived the Hiroshima blast, so they must have some incredible defenses. Then I remembered: cambium. The best metaphor for cambium is the venous system of the human body, roads and pathways that touch every inch of our body delivering life-sustaining nutrients and oxygen. In humans, these pathways deteriorate over time, whether due to age, diet, lifestyle, or simple cellular death. But the cambium in a ginkgo tree, well, in basic terms, it never dies. Within the ginkgo's genetic code there is no "off" switch, or automatic cellular death process.

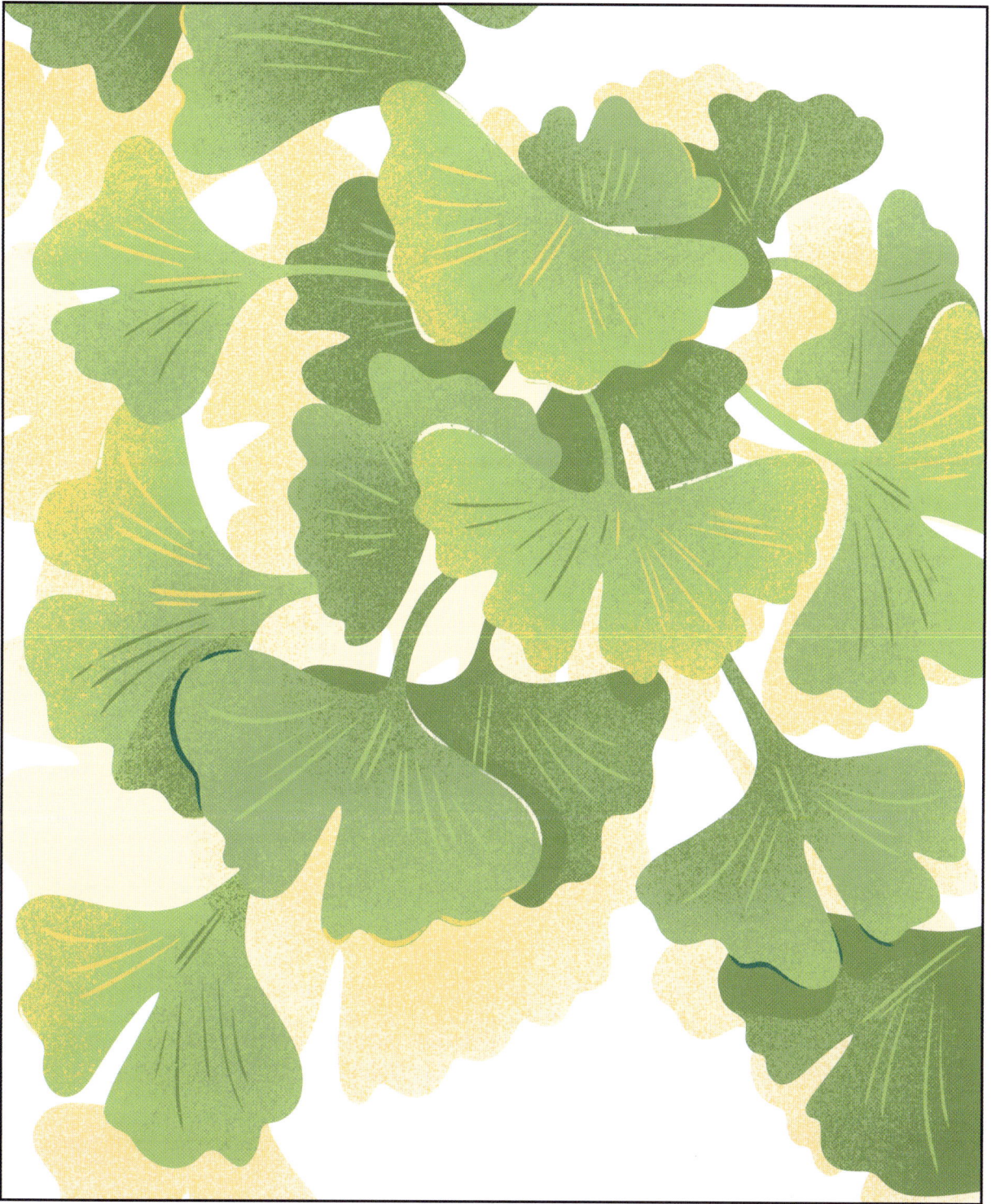

PLANT DATA
USDA hardiness zones: 3 to 9
Water: moderately tolerant of drought, but prefer moist soil
Light requirement: full sun; does not thrive in hot, dry climates
Soil: not picky, prefers sandy soil that is well-drained
Temperature: frost tolerant
Wildlife notes: wild turkeys, pheasants, and woodpeckers like to eat the seeds
Pollinator friendly: wind-pollinating (produces large amounts of pollen in spring)
Pests: relatively resistant, but aphids can annihilate small trees

A hundred-year-old ginkgo keeps right on growing as well as producing natural defenses as if it were twenty.

A single minute under a ginkgo had conjured all these thoughts. It is amazing what simply stopping and pausing for a minute can do. I think this may have been the instant I added "watching leaf foliage turn" to my list of favorite sentiments brought around by fall. And now, every year, many of us wait and watch the thousands of leaves suddenly transition from green to gold, like torches lining the downtown streets of Portland.

If you have the space, go get a ginkgo tree. You will not regret it. In fact, get two, or three, or a dozen. Their golden leaves are so beautiful in fall, you won't even mind the tedious task of raking. They are dioecious and also wind-pollinated, which means you need to have more than one or another one relatively close by for pollination. Both the male and female trees produce flowers, but they look different. The male flowers look like a short cone covered in pollen. The female flower is a solitary stalk about twice as long as the male's with two ovules at the base. The fruit of female trees is known for a strong, rancid butter smell, so seek out males for residential use. The ginkgo's fan-shaped leaves that seem to flutter to get your attention have been represented in art for centuries.

Ginkgo is one of my favorite herbs. I love the papery feel of the leaves and the crunchy sound they make when I blend them into tea formulas. Their smell is slightly sweet, which indicates a nutritive quality. The leaves contain ginkgolides, a compound unknown in any other plant species. Ginkgolides are a class of diterpenoids, which is the scientific way of saying they have both an anti-inflammatory and antimicrobial effect. But they do more than that: they also improve blood flow, protect the central nervous system, and reduce programmed cell death. Reducing programmed cell death (antiapoptosis) in antiaging medicine is a growing area of study.

When I think of ginkgo, I think of its association with increased blood flow. It mainly accomplishes this by relaxing the smooth muscles in arteries, or vasodilation. Think of your arteries like tunnels. Blood and oxygen are flowing through these tunnels to all parts of your body. When you take ginkgo, it makes those tunnels bigger, which means more blood flow and oxygen circulation. This is particularly helpful for the brain. Numerous studies have shown that ginkgo benefits both cognitive thought processing and memory. Research has also focused on ginkgo's use in reducing vascular type dementia and Alzheimer's. If we become more sedentary later in life not only does circulation slow down, but our circulatory system becomes weaker. When we move our body we give our circulatory system a workout as well as a bit of a flush out. This keeps it strong so blood can easily reach all extremities and far-reaching body parts. Moving your body and including ginkgo in your routine will mobilize the ginkgolides to reach throughout your system.

Ginkgo's anti-inflammatory effects have been also researched for intermittent claudication (IC), anxiety, eye health, and its effects on platelet-activating factors. IC is leg pain during exercise because of insufficient oxygen; as a result your muscles can't keep up with the demand and you cramp. Ginkgo's effect on platelet-activating factors can reduce allergies, asthma, and inflammation. GABA, a neurotransmitter that slows us down and promotes a sense of calm is also affected by ginkgo.

I could go on and on here. If you do your own research, you'll find that ginkgo has been around the proverbial research block. When I blend a patient formula, I will put ginkgo in either the main action or nourishing spot. (See the herbal blending instructions in the appendix.) But in all honesty, it could also go in the stimulating spot as it can perform all three actions within a formula.

Ginkgo Recipes

INDICATIONS

- Anxiety
- Allergies
- Depression
- Dementia
- Fatigue
- Headaches
- High cholesterol
- Libido
- Mental fogginess, confusion
- Parasites
- Raynaud's disease
- Stroke recovery
- Tinnitus
- Vision decline

Generally regarded as safe for all populations. Avoid for one week before surgery due to PAF inhibition. Avoid if you have history of seizures or diagnosis of epilepsy. May interact with Xanax and anticoagulants; consult your health care practitioner before combining.

GINKGO BRAIN BARS

Having ready-to-go snacks that are medicinal and healthy definitely make it easier to get through long days. Here is a simple and delicious snack bar for that midafternoon craving.

Items needed:
8-x-8-inch baking pan
Small mixing bowl
Large mixing bowl
Parchment paper

Ingredients:
1 cup smooth nut butter
¼ cup tahini
⅔ cup raw honey
3 tbsp. coarsely ground seed/nuts: sunflower, pumpkin, almond, cashew
2 cups organic rolled oats
½ cup ginkgo leaf powder
1 tsp. vanilla extract
½ cup mini chocolate chips
Pinch of salt

In the smaller bowl, mix together nut butter, tahini, honey, vanilla, and salt. Set aside.

In the large mixing bowl, combine oats, ginkgo powder, nuts/seeds, and chocolate chips.

Fold into the nut butter mixture and continue to mix until cohesive. It may appear dry at first; continue to mix until it's consistently moist.

Line your baking pan with parchment paper and press the mixture into the pan. Use a second piece of parchment paper or a small loaf pan to flatten the bars down.

Chill for 1 hour, then cut and store in an airtight container in the refrigerator.

EYE SUPPORT SYRUP

If I could turn every medicine into a syrup, I would. Luckily, ginkgo and these other helpful herbs blend together nicely for a yummy syrup that is the perfect tonic for eye health. I'm at the stage of life where I cannot deny that my eyes are aging (hello, reading glasses); after using this regularly, my eyes actually improved so much I didn't need lenses anymore for computer work.

Items needed:
Saucepan with lid
Strainer
Stirring spoon
Glass storage bottle

Ingredients:
1 oz. dried or fresh ginkgo leaves
1 oz. dried or fresh bilberries
1 oz. blueberries
10 oz. organic cane sugar

Place all ingredients in a saucepan and add 48 oz. (6 cups) of water. Turn on the heat and bring it to a slow boil. Place the lid slightly ajar, then gently boil down the until it's about ⅓ of the original volume. Double strain it, wash out the saucepan, and return the liquid to the pan. Add 10 oz. of organic cane sugar. Stir until dissolved. Usually you don't need to add more heat, but if the liquid has cooled down significantly, turn the burner on the lowest setting to dissolve the sugar completely.

Pour into a clear bottle and store in the refrigerator. Take 1 to 2 teaspoons per day.

GINKGO MORNING JUMP-START SMOOTHIE

I love a morning smoothie, particularly in the summer when the Oregon berries are bountiful. This easy morning breakfast or mid-morning snack helps my brain, and body, keep going.

Items needed:
Blender or smoothie blender

Ingredients:
½ cup milk of choice: dairy, oat, hemp, macadamia
1 cup water
4 or 5 ice cubes
2 tsp. ginkgo leaf powder
½ cup mixed frozen berries
½ peeled banana
2 tsp. ground flaxseeds
1 tsp. chia seeds

Put all ingredients into a blender and blend for 30 seconds. Enjoy!

GINGKO LONG-LIFE TEA

I do love a cup of tea, and my ginkgo long-life blend is one I drink cold in the summer and hot in the winter. It is a natural pick-me-up and I often visualize how the tea causes extra oxygen and glucose to circulate throughout my body.

Items needed:
Kettle
Mixing bowl
Glass storage jar
Tea strainer and mug

Ingredients:
1 part ginkgo leaf
1 part lemon balm
½ part oatstraw
¼ part dried orange peel
¼ part rosemary leaf

Blend all dried ingredients in a mixing bowl and stir well. Store blend in a glass jar, away from heat. Place 2 tsp. in a tea strainer, pour boiling water over, and steep for 10 minutes.

Hawthorn

Crataegus oxyacantha,
Crataegus monogyna,
Crataegus laevigata

Family: Rosaceae
Parts used: dried berry,
leaf, and flower
Medicinal actions:
astringent, cardiac,
diuretic, carminative,
tonic
Native geography:
Europe, northwestern
Africa, and western Asia

I have a hawthorn at home. It sits on the highest part of our property, where the grass grows tall and bright in the spring. It was one of the first trees on this piece of land that I was drawn to. We moved in in the spring, just when the five-petaled flower clusters had burst forth. Just five months later, I became enchanted with its fruit, known as the haw. Its deep-crimson clusters of red berries are the things of fairy tales, dripping off the tree, beckoning you to them. Hawthorns often grow in relative isolation, but if you scan the horizon near one, you will most likely see others close by.

Some trees are so embroiled in myth, it is hard to escape ascribing a supernatural presence to them when you come across them. Hawthorn is one such tree. Without the cover and protection from hawthorns, how else could fairies travel safely? In Celtic traditions, they are a highly prized tree; anyone who damages or insults one is surely to receive swift punishment. An entire book could be written about hawthorn and its connection to myth, female sovereignty, and the act of deepening one's relationship to oneself. In many myths, the hawthorn represents a goddess, crone, Gaia, or the soul—some sort of cosmic higher being, whichever you choose to recognize. When you first see a hawthorn tree, it might be those scented flowers or the ripe red berries that draw you close—but once you arrive, you have to wade through a thicket of branches lined with sharp thorns to reach them. Pain comes before delight, and the hawthorn has been intertwined with legends involving having to undergo tribulation

to reach a reward or enlightenment. I like to think that hawthorn was created in the spirit of giving, but it reminds us that those who give must be treated with kindness and respect. Learning to navigate around delicate obstacles helps us to grow.

My hawthorn tree is next to my goat barn, so I walk by it twice a day. Developing intimate relationships with nature of the kind you can only make through daily intimacy serves a purpose for me: it fills a very basic innate need for connection. As a doctor, I've read countless studies on the importance of humans having a community and how that plays into mental health. Many studies show that having family, friends, or a specific social network (the live kind) to regularly engage with boosts positive self-reflection and frame of mind. This translates directly into physical health; the body-mind connection matters.

But what is rarely studied and less known is that having a connection with nature can have many of the same effects on mental health. I am often much more satisfied after a day in the woods than I would ever be after a social function, even one among friends. While some people crave conversation, I crave communion with nature. In the mountains, among trees, alongside rivers, at the ocean, I become aware of the vibrational energy nature gives off. It centers me, and allows me to interact with my family and community from a place of authenticity.

Each day, I say hello to my hawthorn. I watch it for the subtle changes that the passing of the seasons creates. I feel like a mother hen, checking for broken limbs and noting, like

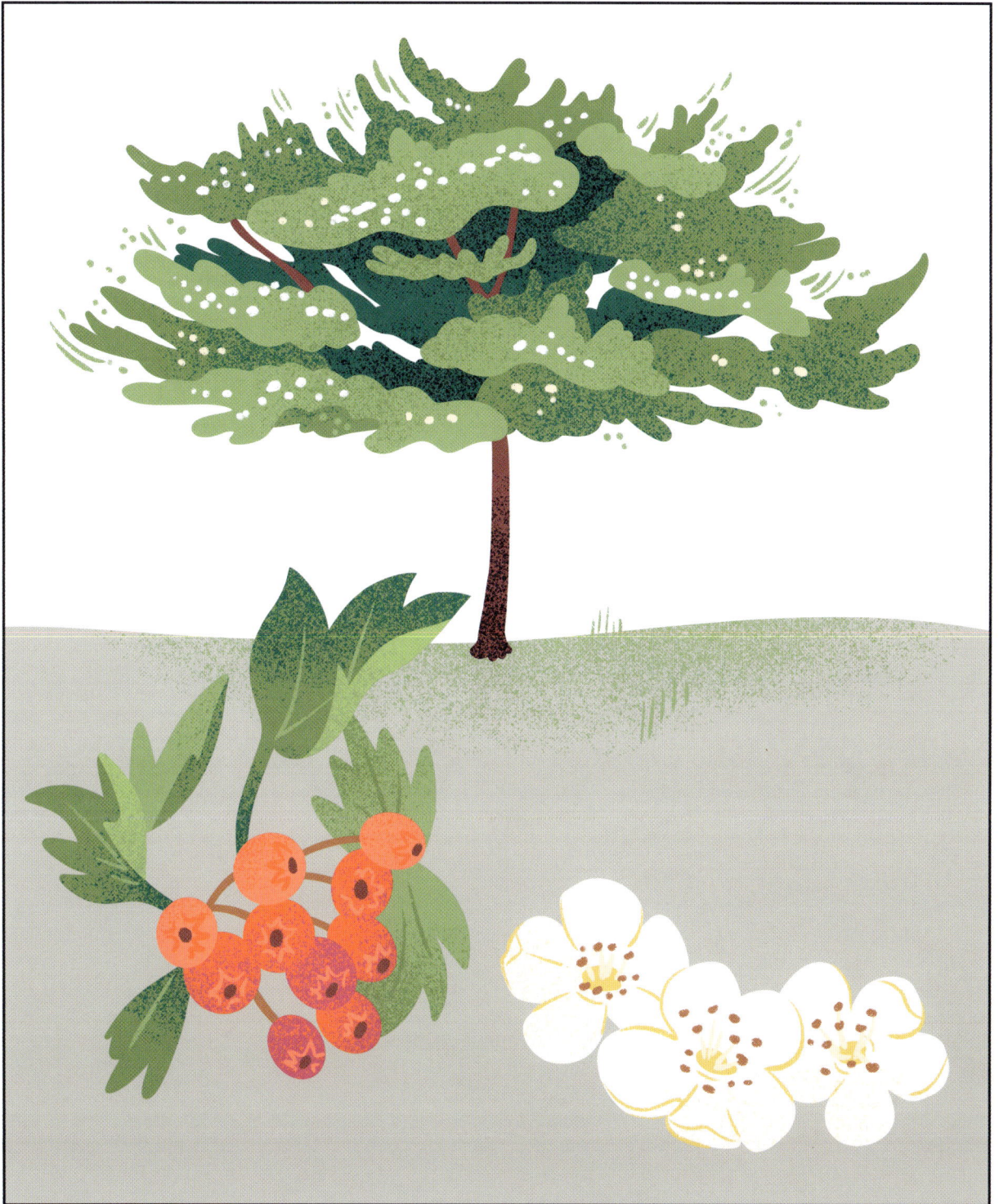

Water: regular watering, especially during the first couple of years after planting to establish its root system; once etablished, it becomes relatively drought-tol-erant

Light requirement: prefer full sun for a mini-mum of 6 hours per day

Soil: not picky, very tolerant of many soils, but does prefer a well-drained area

Temperature: hardy, highly frost tolerant

Wildlife notes: deer and rabbit both love its bark and twigs; a staple for thrushes and waxwings during the winter months

Pollinator friendly: bees, moths, butterflies, and hummingbirds

Pests: aphids, beetles, leafminers, scale insects, spider mites

a scientist, if anything has changed from the previous day. I collect the flowers in the spring and the berries in the fall, and always write down the date of collection so I can track it year over year. I make tea from its products and drink it while leaning on its trunk. I talk out loud, commenting on its beauty or shar-ing my amazement in watching the berries change from bright green to deep orange and finally to a brilliant maroon. And every day as I walk back from the field toward my house, I wonder who really is taking care of whom in this scenario.

———————

The tightly wound flowering buds begin to show themselves in mid-spring, producing clusters of green buds on corymbs. These cor-ymbs often consist of 25 flowers each, making it an incredible display once opened. Flowers are white and have a single pistil and five pet-als; they look similar to wild cherry blossoms, but are often a bit later. Buds typically open in early May. Pollinators love hawthorn, so you'll often see bees and pollinator wasps buzzing joyfully around.

The leaves are alternate, up to 2.5 inches long and have 5 to 6 deep lobes. The stipules are at the base of each leaf. The underneath side of the leaf is lighter than the top, and the new leaf shoots are the brightest of green in color. After the blooming, the tree fills out nicely.

The fruit—a berry—forms in the late spring and fall, depending what zone you are in. They are a beautiful deep red with one seed. They are a major food source for winter birds and dunnocks, blackbirds, thrushes, and finches love them. I wait almost one week after the berries ripen to harvest them, to give them a little time to cure and sweeten up. Nothing scientific about that preference to note, just

one herbalist's experience. Remember not to harvest them all, just take what you need and leave the rest for the wildlife.

Hawthorn is a deciduous tree. Its trunk and fissured bark stands out in winter, and you can see why this irregular, twisted form could have become associated with dark fairy tales at this point. The thorns on the branches are all that will remain throughout winter.

Hawthorn is one of those trees that provides more than one medicine. We use both the leaf and flower as well as the berry. Hawthorn berry is most commonly found in herb shops as well as in formulas designed to support the cardiovascular system. The berry works on the contractility and tone of the heart. Studies show antioxidant effects, lipid-lowering potential, anticardiac remodeling, anti-inflammatory and cardiac toning effects. The leaf and flower are more specific to the overall vascular system, giving it strength and improving integrity. I also reach for the leaf and flower when blood flow is sluggish or there is a propensity for cold hands and feet.

With hawthorn's excellent safety profile, coupled with its lack of herb-drug interac-tion, which has been proven through clinical trials, it warrants being included in most treatment strategies surrounding cardiovas-cular disease, especially in the early stages of disease progression. Cancer, diabetes, high blood pressure, and lipidemia have all reported positive findings with the regular use of hawthorn. Part of the reason is due to its polyphenols, which is a powerful type of antioxidant found in some plants. We are under constant assault from free radicals in both our food and our environment. Antioxidants neutralize free radicals by donating electrons. This, in simple terms, turns the free radical "off."

I also include hawthorn in many of my sleep and antianxiety formulas. While it is not strictly classified as a nervine, I find the vasodilating action to have positive effects on an overly tense person. Combining hawthorn with other nervine herbs, such as hops or skullcap, has proven to be efficient in reducing time needed to fall asleep, reducing frequent waking, and reducing generalized anxiety. Because of its safety profile I also include hawthorn in many of my children's formulas for overactivity, to either calm generalized overactivity or in formulas that are taken after dinner to aid in winding down and preparing for bed. Its gentle nature soothes the slow and nourishes the heart.

Hawthorn Recipes

INDICATIONS

- Anxiety
- Arrhythmias
- Asthma
- Atherosclerosis
- Circulatory disorders
- Congestive heart failure
- Diarrhea
- Gallbladder spasm
- Hyperlipidemia
- Insomnia
- Sore throat, external gargle

Generally regarded as safe for all populations. Species makes a difference with hawthorn: the medicinal varieties Crataegus oxyacantha, Crataegus monogyna, and Crataegus laevigata all have white flowers. Hawthorn has shown to have an effect on the angio-tension converting enzyme; because it can support blood pressure regularity, it is best not to combine it with blood pressure medication. Traditionally, hawthorn was used for digestive conditions such as diarrhea and gallbladder ailments and a go-to gargle for sore throats.

HAWTHORN KETCHUP

Aside from making amazing medicines with hawthorn, you can easily incorporate it into your daily diet, too. Hawthorn jelly, syrup, and muffins are just a few ideas. Since I grew up in the Midwest and A1 sauce was an integral part of almost every meal, I still secretly crave its flavor—just not its sodium. This comes close to that original taste. If I'm going to prepare meat for a meal, I will almost always marinate it. Infusing it with a delicious marinade fills any cut with extra flavor. This hawthorn ketchup works for most meats. I keep it on the table as a condiment, too.

Items needed:
Small Dutch oven
Strainer
Bottle for storage
Sieve
Hand blender

Ingredients:
28 oz. fresh hawthorn berries
1 granny smith apple, chopped
1 white onion, diced
1 lemon, sliced
2 cloves garlic, crushed
1 1-inch piece of ginger, grated
10 oz. apple cider vinegar
10 oz. water
6 oz. light brown sugar
2 tbsp. cumin
1 tbsp. allspice
1 tbsp. nutmeg
2 tbsp. worcestershire
2 tbsp. soy sauce or tamari
1 tbsp. molasses, blackstrap or sweet
½ tsp. salt
pinch black pepper

To begin, clean and stem berries and give them a good rinse in cool water. Add the berries, apple, onion, lemon, garlic, and ginger to the Dutch oven and cover with 4 cups of water. Bring to a simmer and cook for 30 to 45 minutes.

Add the remaining ingredients and simmer, uncovered, for 45 to 60 minutes to thicken. Stir often to ensure you aren't burning the bottom.

Turn off the heat and let the sauce cool for 30 minutes. Then blend it for 30 or 45 seconds, until mostly smooth.

Pass the sauce through a fine sieve to remove all unblended bits and pulp. Adjust seasoning as desired.

Bottle and store in a cool, dark place. Once opened, keep in the refrigerator and use within a few weeks.

HAWTHORN HEART BLEND

Keeping the circulation system vibrant and nourished is something I think about more and more as I age. It's no wonder heart disease is still top of the list of concerns for women over the age of fifty. Women carry a lot of responsibility for their families, communities, and workplaces, which can result in an endless to-do list. This can result in feelings of being constantly overwhelmed. All of this had an impact, physically and emotionally, on the cardiovascular system. I typically spend one month each year focusing on supporting this bodily system specifically, and I use this formula as part of my cardio/circulatory nourishment.

This can be made into a tea, tincture, or syrup.

Items needed:
Tea: mixing bowl and spoon, glass storage jar for tea blend
Tincture: mason jar, strainer

Ingredients:
2 parts hawthorn berries
1 part hawthorn leaves and flowers
½ part gotu kola
½ part bilberry
½ part safflower
½ part fennel seed

Tea
Mix all herbs together. Put the blend into a glass storage jar and label.

To make by the cup: Add 2 teaspoons to a tea strainer and pour hot water over. Let steep, covered, for 10 minutes.

To make medicinal strength: Add 4 tablespoons to a 32-oz. mason jar. Pour hot water over the herbs to the top and let steep for at least 4 hours or overnight. Strain and drink, hot or cold, three times per day.

Tincture
Add all the herbs to a glass jar and pour vodka or apple cider vinegar over. Use just enough liquid so there is approximately 1 to 2 inches of headspace left in the jar.

Close tightly, and label with the contents and date. Keep in a cool, dark place but be sure to shake vigorously, every day, for 2 to 3 weeks. Strain twice and then pour into a storage bottle and label.

CHILDREN'S BEDTIME SYRUP

What child doesn't like a sweet treat before bed? I found this syrup to be a winner with my kids. I would often offer one teaspoon before bed as part of our bedtime routine. It is a combination of hawthorn berries with other botanicals that gently encourage the mind and body to relax into slumber.

Items needed:
Stockpot
Mixing spoon
Strainer
Glass storage bottle

Ingredients:
1 oz. hawthorn berries
½ oz. chamomile flowers
½ oz. rose petals
½ cup honey

Simmer 4 cups of water on medium with the hawthorn berries, until water is evaporated by half. Turn off the heat and add the chamomile flowers and rose petals. Cover for 10 minutes and then strain, twice. Add ½ cup of pure honey while mixture is warm and slowly stir until dissolved. Let cool, then transfer into a glass storage bottle.

Hemlock

Tsuga canadensis,
Tsuga heterophylla,
Tsuga mertensiana

Family: Pinaceae
Parts used: bark,
needles
Medicinal actions:
Bark: alterative, anti-inflammatory, astringent.
Needles: antioxidant,
antiseptic, astringent,
circulatory stimulant,
diaphoretic, diuretic,
immune tonic
Native geography:
North America,
particularly Michigan,
south-central Ontario,
extreme southern Que-
bec, New Brunswick, and
Nova Scotia

The title of the article was "Beware of Bears." I had just picked up the *Crater Lake News* for some evening reading in my tent. It was the newspaper the park ranger had given us with our entrance tickets as we drove through the gate. I love settling in to read in my camp chair once I get camp pitched. Dan, my boyfriend at the time, was a fun-loving guy—albeit a bit young and often distracted—who loved outdoor adventures as much as I did. We'd decided, last minute, to scoot down to Crater Lake for a late-summer getaway.

Crater Lake is approximately 230 miles south of Portland, Oregon, and 400 miles north of San Francisco, California. It's the deepest lake in the United States, a former volcano (Mount Mazama) that erupted and turned into what's technically called a caldera. The peak of the volcano is still intact, but water gradually filled in the crater all around it, creating an island in the center of the lake. It's also famous for "the Old Man of the Lake," a hemlock stump that has been floating there since 1896. But this fella doesn't float like you would expect a log to—rolled horizontally on its side—it floats perfectly upright, as if it were still standing in the forest. Its top four feet of length bob above the surface of the lake, with thirty more feet submerged below. Its density, which has only increased over the decades, has made it buoyant. And it's never been anchored. It sometimes travels as much as three and a half miles around the lake in one day while other times it has remained in place for months. It's great to mull and invent the reasons why it might do this around a campfire at night…

It wasn't just these stories that drew me to this natural wonder, however. There's also the lake's iridescent blue waters, Wizard Island (the peak of the old mountain), and the phantom ship. With words like "wizard" and "phantom" bandied about, how could I not be desperate to investigate? The phantom ship is actually another island formed in a shape that vaguely resembles an old pirate ship—especially when the fog rolls in. Dan and I had been talking about visiting forever, so when a last-minute break in our schedules aligned, we went for it. We weren't experienced campers then, with our fully loaded backpacks at the ready. We took five minutes to think about what we might need and threw it all in the car. At least we remembered the tent. Whatever else we needed we'd figure out along the way. Ah, youth.

We rolled in as the sun was setting, meaning we needed to get set up quickly for the night. We'd read a guidebook on the drive down that recommended heading up Lightning Springs trail to find backcountry campsites. Haphazardly shoving our minimal gear in two backpacks, we parked the car, slung the packs on our backs, followed the signs, and began up a little hill. We walked a ways with the setting sun and eventually came upon two primitive campsites. We honestly couldn't tell if they were available or if the people who might have reserved them just hadn't shown up yet. We didn't want to pitch our tent only to have the reservation-holding party arrive, so we decided to press on deeper into the woods. Soon, we found a beautiful meadow. We navigated to the center of the meadow and

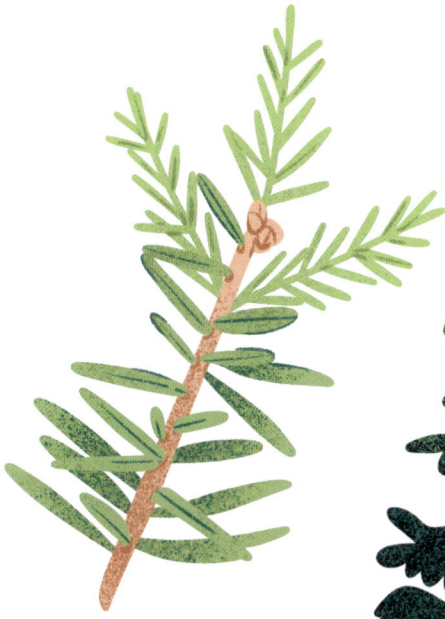

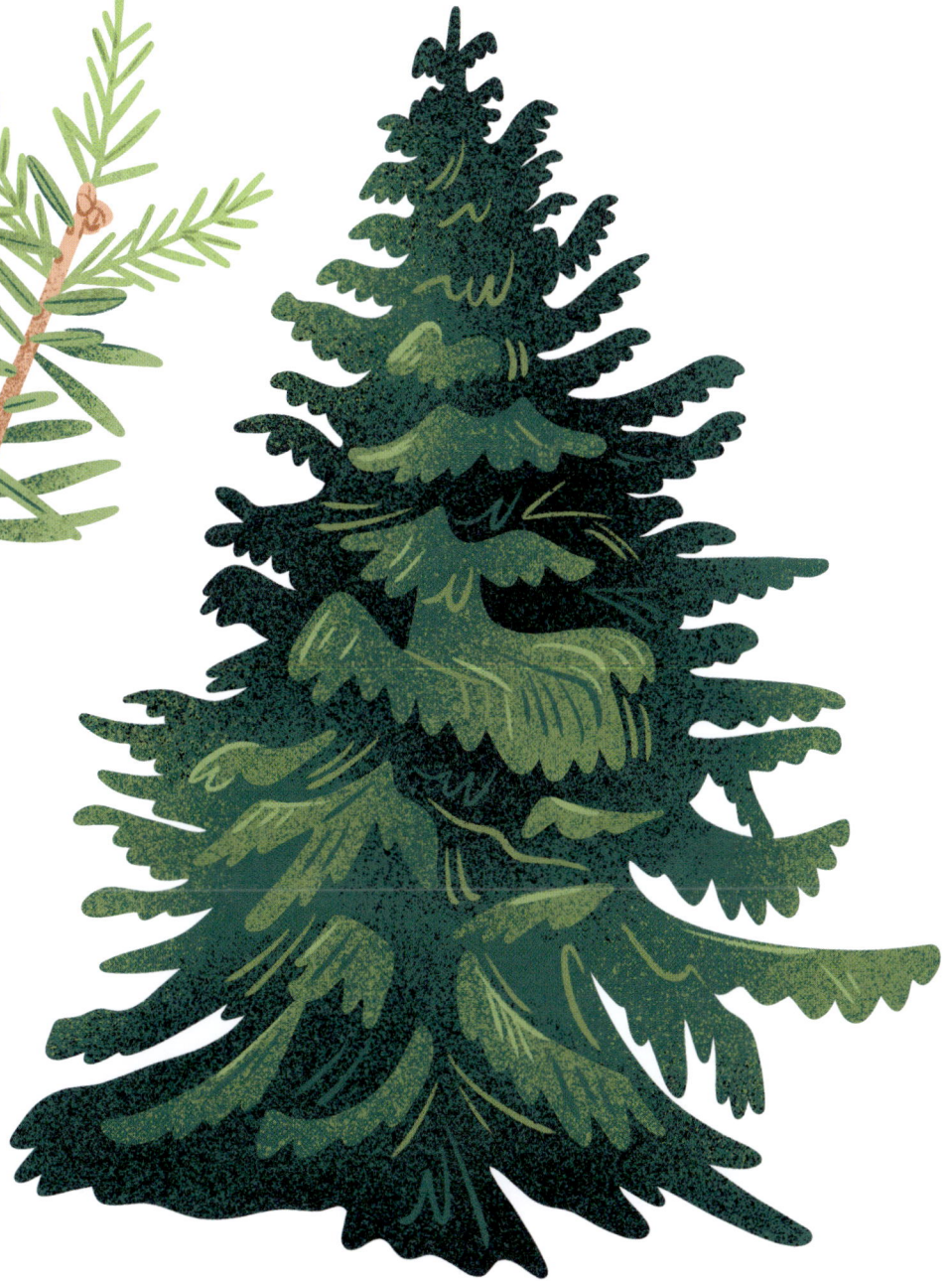

PLANT DATA

USDA hardiness zones: 3 to 7

Water: consistent watering; overwatering weakens root foundations

Light requirement: shade to part sun

Soil: acidic, rocky, cool, moist soil

Temperature: tolerant of cold but not windy areas where soil dries out quickly

Wildlife notes: deer, porcupines, and rabbits use as a food source, and many birds, particularly chickadees and goldfinches

Pollinator friendly: pollinator bats visit regularly

Pests: weakened trees susceptible to hemlock wooly adelgid, scale insects, and loopers, hemlock borer, tip blight, needle rust

began setting up our home away from home for the next few nights. I also began making sandwiches for dinner: tuna fish. I know it's a weird choice, but it was a staple for us at the time and it comes in convenient pouches for camping.

Once my stomach was full, my bed all prepared, I pulled out my headlamp and the *Crater Lake News*, headlined by "Beware of Bears." Bears?!? I could smell the lingering tuna on my breath. I looked at Dan just as he ripped open a very aromatic bag of salmon jerky. We hadn't thought to bring a bear bag—and we'd have to walk a bit to the edge of the meadow to even find a tree. Did we have any rope? Should we put all our food in one of the backpacks and try to hang it from a branch? We debated like this for a while, with one of us trying to convince the other that there were actually no bears and we didn't need to worry about it.

I'm not sure if it was fatigue, laziness, or sheer naïvéte that led us to the decision to put both backpacks in the tent's vestibule—I think we agreed that if a bear did amble by, it would just take the backpack and go. We talked and talked and talked while we lay snug in our sleeping bags, to that point when you know you are beginning to tip into the oblivion of sleep. Right as I acknowledged that, and I mean literally at the exact same time, I heard it. Something taking in smells, short snorts of air. Both of us froze. We were suddenly very awake. A nose pressed up against the tent's thin nylon wall, which in turn pressed against my shoulder. I looked over at Dan; his eyes were the size of saucers, and he was barely peeking out over the edge of his sleeping bag. From deep inside his cocoon he whispered that I should stay still and be quiet. But all I could think about was how that nose reminded me of a kid squashing its face up against glass. I started to giggle. Dan's eyes got even wider, silently pleading

with me to shut up. But I couldn't. Between the funny thought and watching Dan, I exploded in cackles. If I was about to be eaten by a bear due to my own stupidity, I may as well do it laughing.

It turned out not to be a bear. After a few minutes, since the tent was still in one piece, we convinced ourselves to peek out. Well, I convinced Dan to risk his life and look out for the both of us. I secretly had planned an escape route. But, to our surprise, Dan didn't get his face ripped off. In fact, he started laughing loudly. I quickly squeezed out of my sleeping bag and poked my head out. Together, we marveled at the herd of elk that surrounded us. I swear I could hear the Old Man of the Lake laughing at us, too.

As Gary Snyder says, "Plants are all the chemists, tirelessly assembling the molecules of the world." I feel this quote perfectly represents the hemlock tree. There are so many different things going on with hemlock, it only makes sense that it is working to contribute to the greater world somehow. I seek hemlocks when I'm out traveling in the eastern half of the country, and am always sure to harvest some fresh needles for my home medicine cabinet. To me they are one of the most beautiful conifers—whether growing wild or as an ornamental addition around a patio or garden. I always think these tall trees look like a Muppet—a big, goofy furry, droopy tree. The branches slope gently downward, so I always imagine it, at any moment, to come walking toward me, jauntily bouncing up and down. I want to pet the needles once I get up close. They aren't pokey or sharp, but surprisingly soft and calming to touch.

In the spring, the fresh tips (candles) can be harvested and eaten. In Chinese medicine

(CM) spring is the season of the liver, which means it is time to clear out winter accumulations and detox. CM associates sour with the liver, and therefore encourages the intake of sour foods and teas to heal it. Hemlock candles are perfectly sour, which wakes up the liver from its wintry sleep and mobilizes energy. The candles tonify and increase digestive secretions to optimize organ function. Supporting the liver means you are supporting the flow of qi, or the life force of the body—this means physically getting the energy of your body circulating. When you move blood, you move lymph, the garbage collection fluid of the body. When we collect the trash, it opens up pathways and clears organ congestion. All this movement also aids in clearing out old and built-up emotions. Just like the new blades of grass that spring forth from the ground in the spring, our energy awakens and gets released during this time of year.

Later in the season, you can collect and dry the needles for a similar internal effect as mentioned above. More than 60 percent of your immune system is located along the digestive tract; it's worthwhile to dedicate time and energy to keeping it healthy. The use of hemlock can reduce inflammation, improve intestinal tone, and support immunity cells. When the digestive tract isn't busy fighting inflammation—due to poor dietary choices, stress, or decreased function—it can do what it's supposed to do, which is digest food for nourishment and energy and stave off illness.

A great winter medicinal, hemlock needles have an affinity for the respiratory tract. Coughs and colds have a hard time standing up against hemlock's volatile oil content and antitussive action. It is particularly good against a wet type of cough, as it helps to break apart phlegm and alleviate throat irritation. Hemlock needles also are relatively high in vitamin C.

Hemlock Recipes

INDICATIONS

- Atherosclerosis
- Bronchitis
- Cold hands and feet
- Colds
- Cough, particularly the wet type
- Diarrhea
- Digestive complaints
- Joint pain
- Liver tonic
- Mouth ulcers
- Urinary complaints; bladder, kidney
- Wounds

Please don't confuse this with the plant hemlock, Conium maculatum, which is poisonous.

Generally regarded as safe for all populations, but avoid if taking lithium. Tannins may reduce the efficacy of medications taken by mouth.

SPRINGTIME SUPPORT CORDIAL

Cordials have a long history in herbal medicine. They are often referred to as tonics "to warm the heart." Cordials are made with an alcohol base that acts as a solvent to break down the plant cell walls and allow their medicinal constituents to flow into the liquid. Taken in small doses (usually ½ oz.), this recipe is the perfect addition to your late-spring vitalization program. It gets the liver motivated and supports the lower digestive function.

Items needed:
16-oz. mason jar with lid
Wax paper
Glass storage/mason jar

Ingredients:
Hemlock tips (*Tsuga canadensis*)
Alcohol of choice: brandy, bourbon, red wine, or vodka
½ cup organic unrefined cane sugar

The key to good cordials is decent alcohol and a proper flavor pairing. For hemlock, I prefer a high-quality vodka that doesn't mask the hemlock flavor. If you prefer something sweet or fruity, try bourbon or peach brandy.

Harvest hemlock tips as soon as they emerge from their little casings in the spring. They will be bright green and look like tiny, flattened tassels. Cut just the tips off the plant.

Add the sugar to the bottom of the mason jar, then fill the jar with the collected hemlock tips. Next, add your alcohol, filling it to the top.

Place a piece of wax paper over the opening before putting on the jar's O-ring and lid. Shake well. Label with contents and the date. Keep the jar in a cool, dark place, shaking it every day for three weeks. Strain, then store in a clean glass jar, and enjoy!

HEMLOCK SALAD DRESSING

Try this yummy dressing on your next salad.

Items needed:
Food processor
Mixing bowl

Ingredients:
½ cup spring hemlock buds
½ cup good-quality olive oil
¼ cup apple cider vinegar
1 tsp. nutritional yeast
1 tsp. coconut aminos
1 tbsp. honey

Optional: get creative with spices and add oregano, basil, or thyme, to taste

Place the hemlock buds in a food processor. Pulse until finely chopped.
Mix all the remaining ingredients in a small bowl. Then slowly add this to the hemlock buds while the food processor is running on low. Blend just until combined. Enjoy!

Holly

Ilex opaca, Ilex vomica, Ilex aquifolium, Ilex cornuta

Family: Aquifoliaceae
Parts used: roots, leaves
Medicinal actions:
astringent, diaphoretic, diuretic, expectorant, febrifuge
Native geography:
Europe, Mediterranean; holly has adapted to many different environments in the US, with *Ilex opaca* found mainly in the east and *Ilex aquifolium* in the Pacific Northwest and California

Note: the berries of Ilex opaca have historically been used medicinally, but most other varieties are toxic due to saponin content.

If it weren't for the English herbalist Nicholas Culpepper, I would have a hard time finding love in my heart for the holly tree. That sounds a little harsh, and probably isn't quite fair, but despite my best efforts in life I have managed to step barefoot on the piercing leaves of the holly tree more times than I'd like to recall. Before my thirties, when holly trees forcibly interjected themselves into my life, I'd never really noticed them. I had used holly in medicine many times, and I cannot think of the Christmas holiday without thinking of my mom's holly-shaped cookie cutter—always made with green frosting and two Red Hots candies. But I had never seen them growing, much less had them feature in my own home landscape.

The first two I encountered were planted on the corner of a house I rented—right along the driveway, so I would have to squeeze past them to get to my car. They snagged at my coat, my hair, my backpack. Sometimes the leaves would stick to my sweater or jacket without my noticing, until I sat down in my car and was promptly stabbed in the back. In the summer, no matter how wide a berth I gave the trees, a stray leaf would find my bare feet. One time, after I'd cursed holly for the hundredth time, I thought I heard it laughing at me. That's when I started to get suspicious. Was this tree out to get me? Did it watch my movements and strategically conspire with birds and animals to drop its leaves in places it thought I'd walk? I couldn't go more than a day without an attack. It truly felt personal.

At the home I moved to after that, there was a holly tree in almost the exact same spot.

Why were Pacific Northwest landscapers such sadists? I swear I felt it glaring at me as I moved in, as if it knew I already hated it. I decided I needed to remove this negativity from my life, so I decided I would start off on the right foot with this tree. I talked to it, pruned it, kept its base cleaned and fertilized. After all, the winter berries are so pretty, right? It didn't need to know that I mainly did all of this to avoid having any of those dagger-edged leaves fall to the ground where I walked. But I also didn't let the dogs pee on it. I decorated it during the holidays. I was showing good faith. But it didn't care—it poked and stabbed me just the same. No matter how much I swept and raked around its base, leaves found my feet, my hands, my sweaters. I started to secretly give the tree wary side eye as I'd go by, or purposely walk another way to avoid it. If I didn't interact with it, it simply wouldn't have a chance to play out one its devious vendettas. When I eventually moved out, I definitely remember saying "Arrivederci!" I thought that meant goodbye forever, not "Until we meet again."

When I moved into my boyfriend's house, all I could think was, "How in the hell did I never notice that huge holly tree?" The logical part of my brain could understand why people found them appealing—the interestingly shaped evergreen leaves stay colorful in gray winter. But couldn't they be admired from afar, planted far away along a property line? Here, the biggest holly tree I'd lived with yet monopolized my new backyard. (I really should have taken this as a sign the relationship was never going to work.)

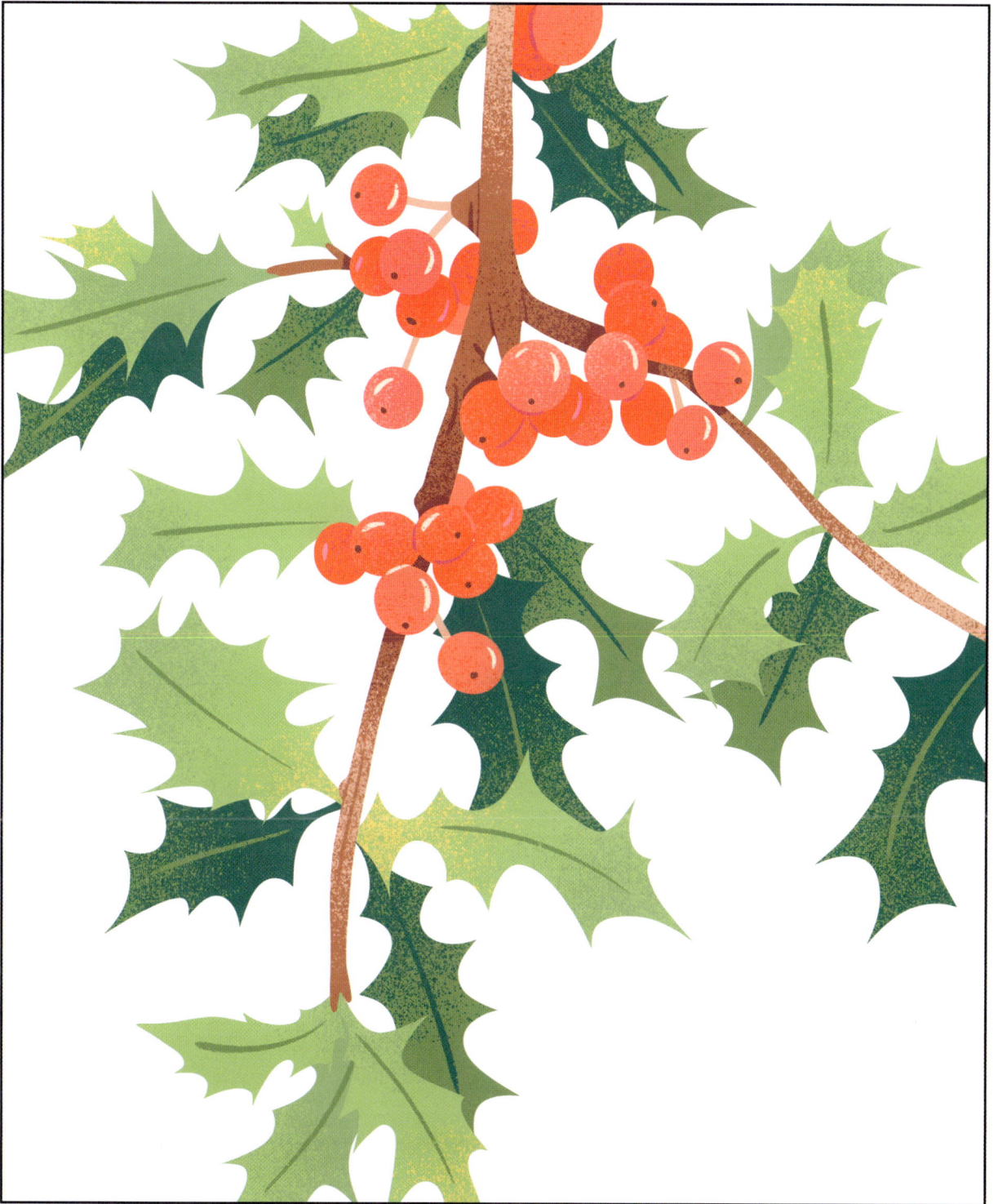

**USDA hardiness
zones:** 5 to 9
Water: water thoroughly
until established; mod-
erately drought tolerant
thereafter
Light requirement:
sun or part shade; avoid
direct hot sun
Soil: loamy soil that is
slightly acidic, moist
and well-draining;
alkaline soil may turn
foliage yellow
Temperature: hardy to
-10˚F, frost-tolerant
Wildlife notes: many
birds eat holly ber-
ries, including robins,
bluebirds, and cedar
waxwings
Pollinator friendly:
important food source
for the honeybee, tiger
and black swallowtail
butterfly
Pests: trees grown
under stress are very
susceptible to root rot

Anyone who knows me knows I'm incapable of killing any living thing. Even mosquitos. Even holly trees that relentlessly attack the most delicate parts of my body and cause exquisite pain. I just can't do it. It isn't my place in the order of things. But when my boyfriend mentioned that the holly tree was growing in a way that was damaging the garage's frame, I secretly smiled. I knew what was coming. He cut that bad boy down, but he'd decided 100 percent of his own accord. My conscience was clear. And as he and our neighbor tackled the task, witnessing the holly's unrelenting lashings against their arms and legs, I gleefully watched from the stoop, drinking my holly leaf tea.

Today, I love and appreciate holly trees—especially those that grow on other people's property.

The three holly varieties I'll mention all have medicinal properties; *Ilex cornuta* has been widely researched and is the species I have had the most experience with personally.

Ilex opaca and *Ilex aquifolium* are found in North America, and both have history with various First Nations. Cherokee tribes used the roots of holly for eye and skin issues by making a fomentation or poultice and apply-ing it to the affected area. The roots are also good at drawing out splinters and insect and snake venom, as well as to address swelling. When my daughter was little, I pulled out a few taproots and boiled them to help her after she twisted an ankle. It was what I had on hand, and it worked remarkably well in reducing the swelling.

Telling holly tree species apart can be tricky, even for me after years of working with them. English holly's leaves will remain glossy even as they mature, whereas the

leaves of the American holly will turn matte. All of them are spiny. They're easy to prune into any shape and if left unattended they will grow into their customary pyramidal form. The small, fragrant, white flowers appear in spring with 4 or 6 petals that are broad with rounded ends and a green center that is bulbous in the female plant and flat in the male. Pollen covers the tip of the male stamens—I always think they look like arms reaching out with an offering.

Holly leaves, considered a cooling agent in Chinese medicine, make a good soak for achy hands and feet. Sometimes when I know I have a long day of gardening ahead, I'll set a bowl of water and mashed-up holly leaves in the sun in the morning. When my work is finally done, I'll relax in a chair and soak my hands for 15 or 20 minutes before hitting the shower.

Chinese Medicine (CM) breaks down the philosophy of healing down to four main categories: meridians, which are like rivers that flow in the body; organs, such as the liver, lungs, and stomach; fluids, including blood, sweat, and tears; and qi, the energy that flows throughout the body. Treatment aims to identify which systems are off balance, and to determine how or why they are being affected. Holly is used in CM to treat the liver, but more specifically "liver heat." When our liver becomes bogged down from overwork (due to spicy foods, excessive meat, alcohol) its function takes a turn for the worse. As the major detoxifier for the body, a decrease in function leads to toxic buildup and the inability to remove waste in a timely manner. This inevitably piles waste on top of waste as the liver falls further and further behind. Just like a car engine revving too high for too long, the internal detoxifying system does the same, leading to heat accumulation. Besides overt digestion issues or skin outbreaks, this also presents as an inability to control anger, grumpiness, feeling hot all the time, and/or pain in the liver area. Holly is one medicinal that can help to correct this disharmony. Just like in Western herbalism, Chinese formulas are blended with plants designed to treat, stimulate, and nourish the patient. Holly would be blended with other herbs to treat liver issues, depending on the overall symptom picture.

Holly Recipes

INDICATIONS

- Arthritis
- Bladder complaints
- Bronchitis
- Congestion
- Fevers
- Gout
- Kidney stones
- Pleurisy
- Rheumatism

*Berries are mildly toxic
 and poisonous to small
 children.

ROASTED YAUPON LEAF TEA

Ilex vomitoria can be cultivated in the garden, but it also grows wild in the southeastern United States. While a relative newcomer to the modern herbal movement, *Ilex vomitoria*, otherwise known as yaupon, is a close cousin to both yerba maté and guayusa; these traditional herbs have been drunk in many cultures due to their natural caffeine levels. Yaupon's caffeine content is similar to green tea, so about ⅓ less than that from a cup of coffee. But, by adding more leaves, you can easily increase its strength. Start by collecting fresh green leaves—just a handful. Once you get the knack of roasting them, collect more at a time and store them in a clean, dry, glass jar for later use.

Items needed:
Pruners
Cast-iron pan
Saucepan
Strainer

Ingredients:
A handful of fresh green holly leaves (*Ilex vomitoria*)

After collection, place the leaves in the cast-iron pan and turn the heat up to medium. Stirring continuously, cook them until they turn dark brown and smell roasted.

Lay the leaves out on a plate to cool, then use your hands to crush the leaves into smaller pieces.

Put three cups of water into the saucepan and bring to a boil. Add the leaves and boil on medium low, for 8 to 10 minutes.

Strain the tea through a fine-mesh strainer, drink, and enjoy.

Feel free to add other herbs such as roasted dandelion or chicory root for a more robust flavor; you can add these after you've boiled the yaupon leaves. After boiling, add ½ tsp of any additional herbs, cover, and let steep for 5 to 8 minutes before straining.

HOLLY LEAF FOOT SOAK

Enjoy this relaxing self-care treatment at the end of a day on your feet. You'll instantly feel rejuvenated and the dogs will stop barking.

Items needed:
Plastic tub or basin, approximately 11 to 12 quarts
Kettle

Ingredients:
1 cup fresh or dried holly leaves
5 drops of an essential oil of your choice: helichrysum, peppermint, or marjoram
1 tbsp. honey

Fill up the basin with hot water, keeping the kettle close by so you can keep adding more hot water as the water in the basin cools down.

Add your holly leaves and the essential oil. Check the temperature to ensure it is not too hot before submerging your feet into the tub.

Relax and enjoy for up to 20 minutes.

Juniper

Juniperus communis

Family: Cupressaceae
Parts used: berries
Medicinal actions:
anti-inflammatory,
antiseptic, aromatic,
carminative, diuretic, expectorant, rubefacient,
stomachic, tonic
Native geography:
Juniper is possibly the
most widely distributed
tree in the world; they
can be found in Asia,
Europe, North and South
America, and Africa

It is the scent that hits me first. I love it, others hate it. Like cilantro. It is a mixture of campfire, smoke, incense, resin, and winter frost. Pungent and very fresh. The groves in eastern Oregon are quite spectacular—thousands of juniper trees grow on the plateaus of Steens Mountain, where cowboys still roam. And in the late summer of 2019, as my kids and I rode horses up the hills in this area, I could smell the juniper scent hanging in the air even before we reached the crest. The junipers were still a couple of months away from producing berries, but the oil on the leaves was enough to infuse our ride with full aroma.

It is said that no two junipers are the same; each stooped and twisted trunk is as uniquely identifiable as a person's face. Juvenile trees start with the perfect conical, Christmas tree shape. But as they grow and age, they take on structural differences that give them distinct personalities. Some turn toward other trees, and some turn away. I always feel when I come up to a group of junipers that it looks as if they were gyrating to music until they realized I was there, then suddenly froze. I always look to see how they mingle with other aspects of nature: one juniper had a split trunk growing around a boulder, embracing the curve and rise of the rock. Sometimes trunks twist so severely they turn back down on themselves and begin creeping along the ground. When I touch the dry, peeling bark, it reminds me of a finger-print whorl—endless unique loops.

While juniper originally grew mostly on rocky slopes with shallow soils and little water, here in the West, as cattle farming moved in and decimated the native grass species, juniper's range began to spread. Birds delight in juniper berries; when they deposit easily-germinated seeds on fertile grazing fields, new trees begin to grow on plains and plateaus.

Our guide on Steens Mountain, John, was the truest kind of cowboy. A man who's worked cattle his entire life and whose life chronicle is recorded as deeply etched lines on his tanned face. He talks slowly, and always with a hint of underlying jest. He tells of the juniper's spread and how as it moves it diminishes the available grazing area. Many ranchers are in a silent battle with juniper. Oftentimes, only they are witness to how and where new colonies pop up year after year. When you have a tree that is drought tolerant, will grow in almost any soil, and is fire resistant, you have a tenacious tree.

As we reached one plateau, John explained just how much the landscape had changed in the last fifty years. We listen to him and the wind, both of which wrap around us and our horses. My son, who is then two but had insisted on having his own horse, is basically tied into the saddle so he can't fall off. As we began to ride, I could see him doubting his choices as he clung to the saddle horn. But John quickly settled his nerves—he'd raised five kids of his own. He'd already won over both of my kids that morning as we all sat and rolled out biscuits for breakfast. He threw scraps from the rounds at the kids when my eyes were diverted, which they instantly devoured like wild beasts. That is why we take these trips. They take us out to the wilderness of Oregon and beyond, yes, but also help us let go of the norms of our daily

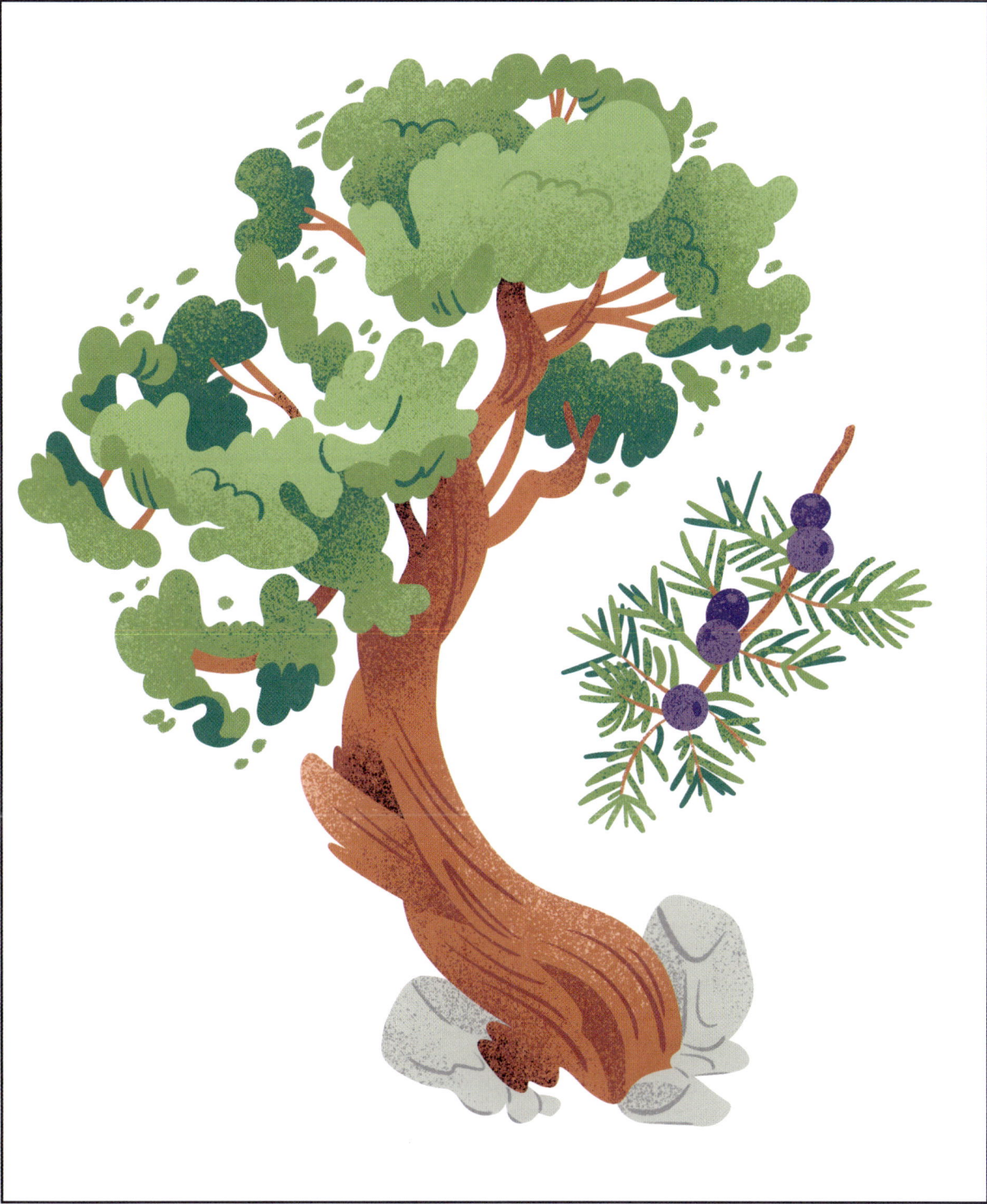

**USDA hardiness
zones:** 3 to 9
Water: allow soil to dry
between waterings to
avoid root rot the first
year; drought tolerant
once established
Light requirement:
full sun
Soil: well-drained
slightly acidic sandy,
clay, or loam soil
Temperature: thrive in
cooler temperatures, but
survive in heat
Wildlife notes: considered one of the top ten
trees for wildlife of many
types. In the colder
months, a single robin
may consume more than
200 berries in a day.
Pollinator friendly:
wind-pollinated
Pests: various blights
and aphids, bagworms,
scale insects, spider
mites

lives and turn us into completely different
people for a few days.

As I looked all around at the plateaus, I
wondered how far the juniper would spread.
The Alvord Desert lay just beyond. Would they
decide to travel that far, testing the boundaries
of their resilience? I wasn't really looking for
scientific answers to my questions that day, but
I did know one thing: I hoped and prayed that
no one would ever stop me or my kids from
roaming as far as we wanted to go.

Junipers are tough trees. Once established,
they seem to cling to existence even in
drought and have been known to live for up to
700 years. It takes three years before a young
tree will produce a harvestable crop of berries.
The first year, it flowers. The second, it'll
produce a hard green berry. In the fall of the
third year, a bright blue berry arrives. Juniper's
berries are sweet, sour, and pungent all at the
same time. A potent medicine, they should
only be consumed for short periods of time
and for a specific purpose.

Junipers are one of the best diuretics we
have available. Many herbalists recommend
juniper in times of bladder or kidney infection, but this is actually not the ideal use of
juniper berries—they have an affinity for cold,
wet conditions of the body and are not recommended during acute stages of infection.
Kidney issues can lead to an accumulation of
stones for various reasons, and when these
stones and gravel are not able to pass you can
get blockage. This can be an acute situation
and lead to excruciating pain, but often
before that happens water accumulates in the
lower extremities and there's pain in the back
around the kidneys. This would be the correct
time to consider juniper. When something
in the body that was designed to move liquid
is blocked, like fluid from the bladder, you'll
typically have a stagnation of fluids and a
buildup of heat. Juniper berries work to dilate
blood vessels and improve fluid flow.

Taking juniper berries as a tonic from
time to time to keep the channels in the bladder and kidneys open and reduce the risks
of congestion is an appropriate use. Or it
can be used after an active infection or stone
attack has passed, to support the system for
long-term health. The one exception would
be to take juniper at first inkling of a bladder
infection; drinking a juniper-based tea for

one or two days can halt its onset by allowing the juniper berries to bind toxins and allow its antibiotic-like action to thwart infection.

Juniper can be used in similar ways for other parts of the body. I've used it for the respiratory system when excess mucous and phlegm are present, edema of the lower extremities, and to support a heart over-burdened by kidney insufficiency. I learned from herbalist John Lust that small amounts can also be given before eating to support healthy hydrochloric acid levels for proper digestion. They are also helpful with digestive infections and cramping. I've found formulas made with juniper to be supportive for PMS and menstrual cramping as well. Dr. John Christopher, one of my favorite American herbalists, used it as a counter-irritant to strengthen the brain, and I'm currently studying how the essential oil acts on recurring headaches.

Juniper Recipes

INDICATIONS

- Back pain
- Bladder complaints; chronic infection, retention of urine
- Colic in adults
- Coughs
- Delayed menstruation from cold environment or exposure
- Eczema
- Edema
- Fever
- Heart burden due to edema or kidney issues
- Headache
- Insect bites
- Joint pain
- Kidney complaints
- Leukorrhea
- Loss of appetite
- Menstrual cramps

Only use dried berries. Speak to your health care practitioner before use if you have heart or kidney disease. Do not use during pregnancy. Juniper may interact with diuretic and diabetic medications.

WILD YEAST STARTER

Juniper berries are a great base for any wild yeast starter to use in making carbonated drinks such as tepache, for beer, and of course for bread. A wild yeast starter consists of a combination of yeasts and bacteria that is created by fermentation, and it will often bring more complexity to the flavor of whatever you are making. Juniper berries work well as a base for a starter because they often already have a yeast bloom on them at harvest time—the white, dusty-looking powder on the berries.

Items needed:
32-oz. glass mason jar
Fermentation top for jar

Ingredients:
½ cup fresh juniper berries
½ organic cane sugar
1½ cups water

Put the berries in the clean glass jar and set aside. Next, combine the sugar and water and stir until dissolved. Add the sugar water into the mason jar with the berries and place the fermentation top on the jar.

Store in a warm, dark place, but stir it several times a day. You should begin to see bubbles forming around the juniper berries around day two or three, with an obvious accumulation by day five. Smell the starter over this period as well; if it smells foul instead of yeasty, discard the mix and start over.

If you use your starter often, you can leave it at room temperature with a towel simply laid over the opening. If you don't use it as much, store it in the refrigerator. It will still require regular feeding. If left at room temperature, feed once every other day. If kept in the refrigerator, feed weekly.

JUNIPER WELLNESS BATH SOAK

I am a strong believer that baths are very underappreciated in our society. They promote calm, relaxation, release muscle tension, and promote restorative sleep. I love a bath that fizzes and smells good—making sensory elements part of the experience will make us want to take more baths, right?

Items needed:
Mixing bowl
Mixing spoon
Mortar and pestle
Storage container for final product

Ingredients:
3 cups Epsom salt
2 cups baking soda
1 cup citric acid
1 cup juniper berries, crushed with a mortar and pestle
¼ cup grapefruit peel
¼ cup apricot oil
20 drops lemongrass or tangerine essential oil

First, mix the Epsom salt, baking soda, and citric acid together.

Add in the crushed juniper and grapefruit peel.

Drizzle in the apricot oil next, mixing with a spoon or your hands until well blended.

Drop in the essential oil and stir a few times to mix.

Transfer the bath salts to a storage container of your choice. In general, glass is preferred for storing herbal preparations, but around the bathtub plastic may be a good choice.

Add 1 cup to the tub as it's filling.

Larch

Larix occidentalis,
Larix decidua

Family: Pinaceae
Parts used: bark,
needles, resin
Medicinal actions:
adaptogen, alterative,
antiseptic, astringent
Native geography:
appears throughout the
temperate mountainous
zones of the Northern
Hemisphere; in the US
they are common in
the subalpine areas of
Montana, Idaho, and
Washington's Cascade
Mountains

It caught my eye immediately. There was something familiar about the tree I was looking at: long, sweeping branches that curved down and slightly back up. I'd seen another just like it almost a year previously, when I had moved to Bellingham, Washington. At almost one hundred feet tall, it staked a serious claim in the backyard at my friend Linda's house. In the summer, it cast glorious shade that provided a place to hide on midday lunch breaks. I'd sit and marvel at its needles that grew in spiky clusters of thirty to forty. You would have expected them to be prickly and sharp, but they were soft and easily folded under the pressure of my touch. Their surprising suppleness made me want to stroke them over and over. I love it when a tree surprises me. In the fall, I had watched that larch turn a beautiful yellow that seemed to radiate like a halo of light. It offered a beacon of brightness that drew the eye.

Before Bellingham, I'd been living in Seattle with the intention of starting graduate school. I moved from Nebraska to Seattle knowing no one and had rented a studio apartment off Craigslist because it had a Murphy bed like in *Laverne and Shirley*. I had applied for one job before I drove out, sending my resume via fax machine. It must be true what they say about a bird pooping on you being good luck, because that happened to me on the way to the interview and I got hired. Between working as a photography librarian at the *Seattle Times* and bartending at a local Irish pub, I was finally making enough money to pay off student loans and credit card bills. When the time came to start my graduate program, though, I realized that as much as I wanted the degree, I wasn't interested in the stress of accruing more debt. I was twenty-six and had little other direction, but I did have a growing realization that the big city would soon swallow me up into its vortex of nightlife. I knew I had to get out and get my head on straight.

And that's how I ended up in Bellingham. I explored the entire state of Washington because I didn't want to retreat back to Nebraska and I felt there was still a lot to see. I visited the Olympic and the Cascade Mountains, wondering if a stint of isolation might be cathartic. I thought about Wenatchee and Olympia and even the Bavarian-style town of Leavenworth. But I ended up falling in love with Bellingham, a hardworking town on the bay. I found a studio apartment on the ground floor of a beautiful Victorian house for $285 per month. Place to sleep, check. Next task was to get a job. All that driving had given me a lot of time to contemplate. I knew I had one thing I was ready to focus on: herbal medicine. Herbal shops where I myself had found help in the form of medicine, resources, or community had always felt safe and welcoming to me. I'd been building my home herbal medicine cabinet for a while, and my brain itched for more. I pulled out the Yellow Pages and was pleasantly surprised to see Bellingham had one herb shop—and it was not too far from my new home. On one of those perfect September days I hopped on my bike and rode along the bay and into downtown. Along the way, I passed a small park with a giant larch tree. Its branches were

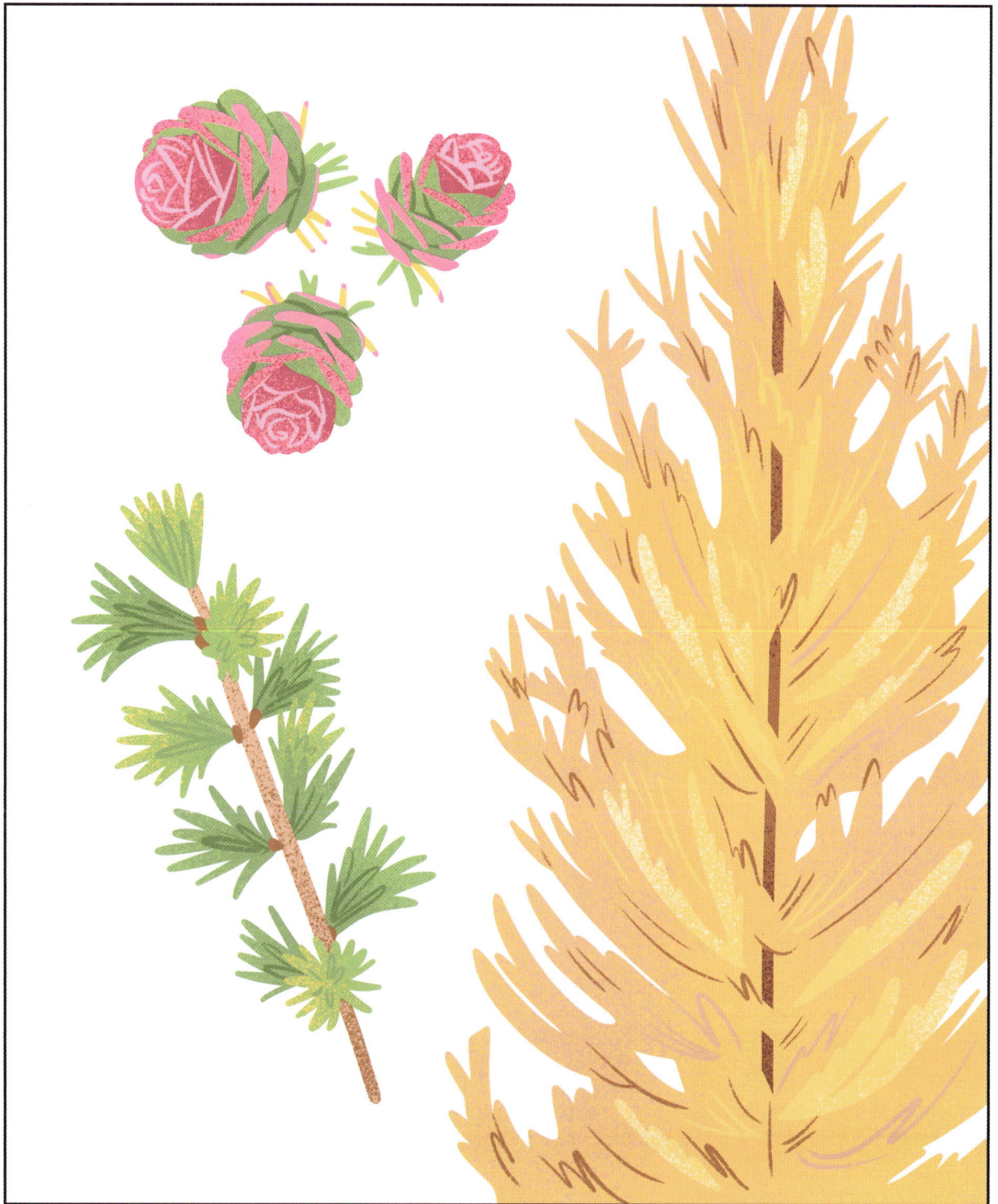

**USDA hardiness
zones:** 2 to 6
Water: keep moist
but not waterlogged,
doesn't like dry soil
Light requirement:
sun to part shade
Soil: well-drained,
slightly acidic loamy soil
Temperature: thrives in
cold, hardy to -45˚ F
Wildlife notes: osprey,
bald eagle, and Canada
geese like to make their
nests up high; bears
find the bark good for
climbing
Pollinator friendly:
early pollen attracts
honeybees
Pests: larch case-bearer,
larch sawfly, rust fungus

swaying in a gentle, cool breeze, waving as if trying to get my attention. Its fall foliage was lit up like a torch. Stopping to acknowledge when something makes us feel a certain way is one of my favorite things to do; but I am a recovering "hurrier," and I constantly have to remind myself that it's okay to slow down to appreciate small-but-rich daily experiences. And stopping to notice a larch in fall is always worth it: this moment doesn't last forever because they are deciduous conifers and drop their needles in winter.

Wonderland Tea & Spice was a cute and unassuming shop with a glass storefront and a big wooden sign above the door. As I walked in, the smell hit me first: a strange and wondrous combination of marshmallow, grandma, and mint. It cast an instant spell of relaxation over me. Next, I spotted an entire wall of glass jars filled with herbs. It took everything in me not to simply open and start smelling each one. As it turned out, Linda, the owner, was there the day I went to visit. I timidly asked questions, and she asked me if I was new in town. After an hour of us chatting away, she offered me a job. I felt like I'd won the lottery.

I might have stayed there forever. I loved the customers, organizing the herbs, and weighing out small bottles of essential oils. But after a couple of years, Linda came in one day and simply said, "I think it is time for you to go." My naive mid-twenties brain at first thought she meant it was time for my lunch break or to do the bank run. But what she was trying to say was that it was time for me to spread my wings. She ultimately propelled me to move my life forward.

I decided to enroll in naturopathic school. My first year, while I was working in the clinic's medicinary, I came across a powdered larch supplement. My mind was instantly flooded with memories of Bellingham, Linda, and the two larch trees I'd

gotten to know there. I'd worked all around Linda's larch tree in her garden, harvesting medicinal herbs and making medicines in her workshop. Yet we had never once discussed larch as a medicine. Maybe it was the soft needles or the golden light it radiated in the fall that drew me to first investigate larch's medicinal qualities. It was this tree, despite my relationships with so many others, that first drove me to study tree medicine. But secretly, I believe it was the wild waving of its branches that got my attention, like a friend gesturing across a crowded room. I still search it out every year to mark the closing of summer, and the ushering in of hot drinks, fireplaces, and cozy blankets.

————

Larch works wonders for gut and immune health. Explaining why means putting on my scientist hat. Arabinogalactan is a starch-like chemical that's found in many plants. Basically, it consists of one giant, highly branched polysaccharide. Polysaccharides are carbohydrates that are well known for their high nutritive value. They work directly on the immune and digestive systems to improve function by increasing response. What that means is that your immune system will be more responsive to foreign invaders, and your digestive tract will increase production of "good" gut bacteria. Plant polysaccharides are also soluble fibers, which, in my opinion, are something we all need more of in our diets. The structure of this polysaccharide has a backbone of galactan and side chains of two sugars: arabinose and galactose. They work as a team, slowing digestive function for more nutrient capture and generating energy production and storage for later use. Specifically, larch arabinogalactan targets "bad" gut bacteria for removal and stimulates the prebiotics of the digestive lining, such as bifidobacteria and lactobacillus. These prebiotics also sometimes increase the release of anti-inflammatory cytokines and inhibit the release of inflammation.

Larch is supportive to the immune system by making it more responsive—notice I did say it *stimulates* the immune system. Unlike echinacea, which turns on the immune system by significantly stimulating the circulation of white blood cells, larch works more like an adaptogen. My teacher Rosemary Gladstar defines adaptogens best: "A group of herbs that have a long history of promoting longevity and increasing the overall strength and resiliency of our bodies." I often refer to their medicinal action as creating balance in the body. They lift up what is down, and they lower what is high. Larch optimizes organ function.

One of my favorite parts of the larch is the female cone, known as a larch rose. Approximately five to eight months after pollination, a small, erect cone will emerge on the branch. Young cones are purple-red and incredibly intricate. They contrast beautifully with the bright green shoots of new-growth needles. Male cones appear as clusters of yellow anthers on the underside of shoots. After ripening, male cones will turn the typical brown color and, once mature, can remain on the tree up to three years.

I often give larch to patients who seem to get every cold that walks through the door. Clinical studies have shown decreases in cold and respiratory infections in participants who take larch for six months, from October to March, when respiratory illnesses are most prevalent. I've also suggested it when a patient presents with digestive complaints that aren't specific to one condition. Recently, cancer studies utilizing larch to support depressed immune function caused by other treatments and studies researching whether larch triggers natural killer cell reactions to target specific cancers have been getting attention.

Larch Recipes

INDICATIONS

- Colds
- Cough
- Digestive health
- Ear infections
- Flu
- HIV/AIDS
- Immune tonic
- Wound healing

*Generally regarded as safe for all populations. There is uncertainty regarding interactions for patients with auto-immune pathologies. Do not take before or after planned organ transplant surgeries.

LARCH SHORTBREAD

Incorporating larch wherever I could was, for a time, an obsession of mine. I love the bright tang of fresh larch needles, so it was fun to experiment. The TV show *Ted Lasso* was airing at about the same time, a source of joy and much-needed escape from the realities of what our world was going through. If you've watched the show you'll know that the main character brings his boss buttery biscuits (shortbread) every morning. See where this is going? Shortbread is absolutely one of my favorite treats. It has a ridiculous amount of butter, but I justify that by adding herbs to make it "healthy."

Items needed:
Mortar and pestle
Stand mixer or hand mixer
Several mixing bowls
Parchment paper
9-x-9-inch baking pan

Ingredients:
2 tbsp. dried larch leaves
1 cup unsalted butter, room temperature
¾ cup powdered sugar
2 cups all-purpose flour
1 tsp. vanilla extract
¼ tsp. salt (optional)
1 egg (optional)
¼ cup organic caster sugar

Using a mortar and pestle, grind 1 tablespoon of the larch leaves until almost a powder and set aside. Next, grind the remaining larch more coarsely, leaving tiny bits of larch leaves intact. Set this in a separate bowl.

Using a mixer, beat the room-temperature butter on high speed for 3 to 5 minutes. Turn the mixer to low and gradually add in the powdered sugar until combined. Stop and scrape the sides from time to time if necessary.

In a separate bowl, sift the flour. Add the vanilla, salt, and finely ground larch needles. Once combined, add this to the butter/sugar on low, mixing just until blended.

Next, line your pan with parchment paper. Transfer the biscuit batter to the pan and spread or pat it in evenly. Refrigerate for 1 hour.

Meanwhile, preheat the oven to 300° F. Next, mix up the topping. Combine the caster sugar and remaining larch needles, stirring to blend. Whisk the egg to create a wash for the top of the biscuits. Brush it across the top, then sprinkle the larch sugar on top.

Score the dough into 16 bars before baking.

Bake for approximately 45 to 60 minutes, on the middle rack, until golden brown. Let cool completely before serving.

PICKLED LARCH ROSES

Try pickled larch roses for a fun and unique—and incredibly delicious—way to bring larch into your daily routine.

Items needed:
Saucepan
Stirring spoon
16-oz. mason jar

Ingredients:
2 cups larch roses, or enough to loosely fill your jar
½ cup vinegar: apple cider, white wine, or white distilled
½ cup water
5 tbsp. organic cane sugar
Pinch of salt
Pinch of black or pink peppercorns

In the saucepan, bring the water, vinegar, and sugar to a boil. Stir often to help dissolve the sugar and protect it from boiling over. Turn off the heat once dissolved. Add the salt and peppercorns and allow to cool.

Pour this pickling liquid over the larch roses in the mason jar, ensuring the liquid completely covers the larch. Cover with a lid and put the jar in the refrigerator for 4 to 5 days before sampling.

Store pickled larch roses for up to 6 months.

Laurel

Umbellularia californica

Family: Lauraceae
Parts used: leaves, seeds
Medicinal actions: analgesic, antirheumatic, nervine, stomachic
Native geography: southwestern North America, western California, and Oregon

The house in front of me didn't look like the photo that had been posted in the Craigslist ad. The house in the photo was blue; this house was yellow. Also, there was a giant tree looming in the backyard that had not been in the photo—how old was that shot? I had showed up an hour early to the showing for this rental. I desperately needed a house, and finding a rental at the time was ridiculously difficult. Portland was a housing nightmare. People had even taken to writing unsolicited letters to owners, trying to persuade them with endearing facts about themselves why they, of all the applicants or offers, should be chosen. That era had ended, and the market had entered a phase of cut-throat and aggressive renting/buying tactics. I wasn't good at outmaneuvering others by conniving design, so I went with the "maybe-if-I'm-first-in-line" approach. As the showing time neared, cars began edging in closer and closer on the street—you would have thought a drag race was about to start. It was pretty apparent who the rental agent was. He had a file of poorly organized rental agreements trailing behind him as he went to unlock the door. With that simple turning of the key, the race began. Like bees escaping from a hive, all of us streamed from our cars and made a mad dash for the front door. I'd barely done a single lap through the 900-square-foot house before I approached the agent to ask what the decision process entailed. "The first one who submits the application to the office wins," he said. Well, I raced home to print, fill out, sign, and submit my application. I even called the rental office to ensure they had received it and

so I could get verbal confirmation of my first-to-submit speediness.

When I finally took a breath, I had two thoughts. One was, "What in the heck is all over the bottom of my shoes?" The second was, "I really didn't even see the entire house. What were the bedrooms like? Was there a backyard?" I was a single mom of a four-month-old and two dogs, and while our needs were minimal, having a backyard for all of us was definitely something on my want list. I knew the open house was over by that point, so I decided to drive back over and see if I could look around. I knew the house itself was vacant, but I still worried about what the neighbors would think as I nonchalantly walked around the front of the house peeping in windows and doing my best to see through closed miniblinds, the hallmark of many rentals. But the back of the house, and therefore the bedroom windows and backyard, weren't accessible from the front or sides of the house. It appeared you either had to go through the garage to get to the backyard or through a series of raspberry brambles that stymied me from my covert mission.

That's when I got the brilliant idea to crawl up onto the recycling bin to try and see into the backyard from the garage side. It was almost dusk, which wasn't helping. A long, tall hedgerow of *Prunus laurocerasus* was annoyingly blocking my view. I was contemplating hopping over the fence when I heard a noise. A scrambling of sorts, and then branches of the hedge rustling. Before I even had time to think, a man's face appeared in the middle of it and said, "Hello." I immediately felt

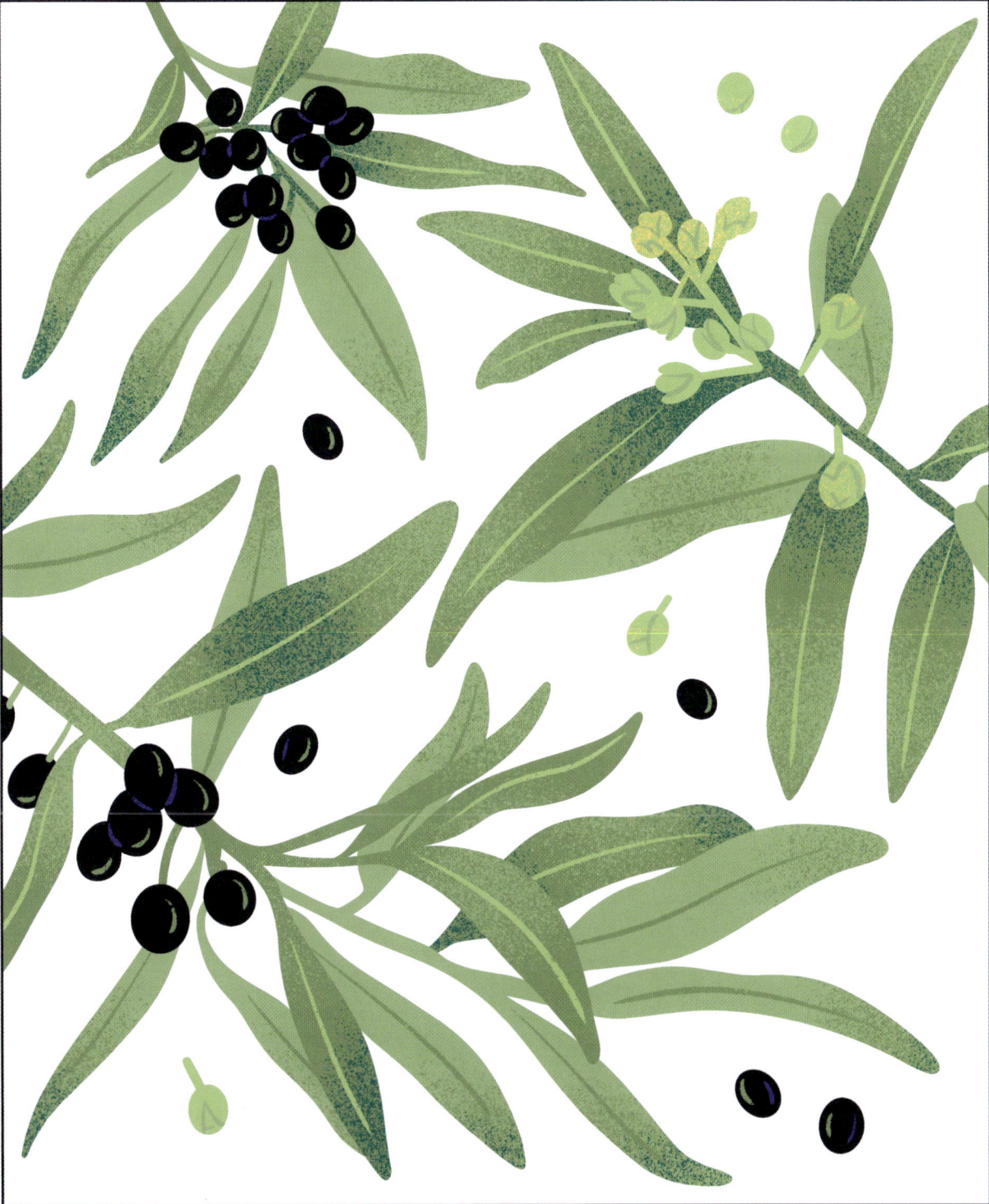

PLANT DATA

USDA hardiness zones: 7 to 10

Water: water heavily when young, requires less and less once established

Light requirement: prefers some shade in warmer climates

Soil: can tolerate sandy, loamy, and clay but prefers it to be moist and well-drained

Temperature: Intolerant of frost

Wildlife notes: black-tailed deer eat the leaves because of moderately high levels of protein; squirrels like the seeds

Pollinator friendly: all pollinators are drawn to this tree for its pollen and nectar

Pests: aphids, white flies, sudden oak death, and heart rot

myself blushing. I was peering into the face of the man who might be my new neighbor, into his backyard. "Hello," was all I could muster initially, but then the word vomit came spilling out about my situation and how I was just trying to get a better understanding of the house and its amenities.

"Well," he said, "I guess I'm glad it wasn't racoons getting into the garbage."

"Nope," I said, "just a crazy person who might be your neighbor." I smiled and said "Yayyyy," and raised my hands like he was winning the best prize of all.

Fortunately, that incident didn't involve the police or a call to the property management company. The neighbors turned out to be incredible. That yellow house turned out to be a saving grace, allowing me and my little family to ground and grow in all the right ways. When I finally got into the backyard I was able to get up close to the tree I'd seen: a mammoth California bay laurel. I had to step back just a bit and lean way back in order to see all the way to the top. On warm days, it emitted a fragrance of cardamom and nutmeg on the breeze that came right into our bedroom windows. It dropped bon bons, too—a hard little nut that I tried to make coffee out of but quickly realized they were nuts best left for the squirrels. And as for the bottom of my shoes, they were permanently stained from its fruit.

———————

I had never really used California bay medicinally before, so I was excited to learn everything I could about it since I suddenly had an endless supply of leaves. Limited specific research is available, but it has been shown to have the capability to reduce and in some cases eliminate MRSA and gram-positive types of bacteria. MRSA is a staph infection on the skin that is antibiotic resistant. It appears as a red, swollen, and eventually infected rash on the body. Laurel has a chemical profile of quinones, alkaloids, flavonoids, cardenolides, tannins, and saponins—all help reduce infection. This was good to know, but I wanted to learn ways I could use it in my day-to-day routines as well.

I knew that the leaves can be used for a variety of conditions, so I started using myself as a guinea pig. One resource mentioned its use as a tea for sore throat and cold with stuck phlegm. Here in the Pacific Northwest, that is a very common cold type. Within months, I was able to test it out. The oils in the leaves make for a yummy tea, but best if only steeped for a minute or two. It feels a bit stimulating, and the aromatics produce a slight numbing action on the throat. I found it to be both soothing and invigorating to the respiratory tract.

Another resource had mentioned its ability to ease digestive bloating. One evening after a bit of overindulgence, I decided to give it a try in place of my usual digestion blend. Surprisingly, it worked quite quickly at dispelling the overfull and distended feeling. Research has shown consistent positive results with its use for the reduction of intestinal cramping and gastroenteritis.

As I alluded to above, the seed is prolific but truly a hard nut to crack. It is a laborious task to retrieve the useful "meat" from inside, but apparently it does have a long history of use. At one point I read that there is a small amount of caffeine in them, so I tried to collect enough to make a coffee substitute. I gave up pretty quickly, but the one cup I did harvest enough to make was definitely stimulating and had the aroma and slight flavor of chocolate.

The ground meal from the seed has traditionally been used to treat cold sores. It can be collected, ground, and used as a flour for baking breads. The leaves can be used as a bay laurel substitute in soups and stews—but use half of the amount because it is much stronger.

The California bay laurel is an evergreen tree of considerable size. While the average height is 40 to 80 feet, many reach heights of 100 feet or more. It is evergreen, which makes it a pleasant addition to most landscapes. It flowers in April, and the seeds ripen from October to November. It is a hardwood that is much prized due to the beauty of its grain; this feature also gives it a strong resistance to most types of insect attack. With the high volatile oil content of the leaves, I believe it naturally creates a certain level of antiviral activity within the space where it lives. Just leave your windows open to get the gift of clean, virus-fighting air.

Seedlings can be fragile, so it is best to allow them to grow in a greenhouse their first year. Plant them out into their permanent positions in late spring or early summer the following year, after the last expected frosts.

Laurel Recipes

INDICATIONS

- Colds
- Cough
- Digestive complaints
- Flu
- Nervousness
- Neuralgia
- Pain
- Rheumatism
- Stress
- Wound healing

*Can cause skin sensitivity and rashes with some populations. The aromatic oils are strong and if inhaled deeply can cause headache and dizziness, and allergic reactions for some

SOOTHING BATH SALTS FOR RHEUMATISM
Please ensure you do not have an allergy or skin sensitivity to California bay laurel before use

After a long day of gardening, there is nothing like a nice, long bath. Next time, add this bath salt combination for a muscle-relaxing experience.

Items needed:
Mixing bowl
Mixing spoon
Storage container or glass jar
Large muslin bag

Ingredients:
1 cup California bay laurel leaves
1 cup chamomile flowers
4 cups Epsom salt
20 drops of lavender or orange essential oil

Mix the California bay laurel leaves with the chamomile flowers, then add in the epsom salt. Once it is all mixed together, drop in the essential oil and stir. Transfer to your storage jar.

Add 1 cup to a muslin bag and submerge it in the bath. Relax and enjoy. Best before bed.

ROASTED LAUREL NUTS

Harvest laurel nuts as soon as they begin to fall, and process them immediately after. You want them to be ripe, which means they should feel a little soft. If they aren't soft(ish), let them ripen for a few days on your kitchen counter. This makes it much easier to peel away the reddish-purple outer layer.

Lay the nuts on a cookie sheet and dry them in a convection oven at 300° F for 10 to 15 minutes, or just until the nuts begin to crack open. Allow to cool, and pull the nut from each bon bon.

Then turn up the heat to 400° F and roast the nuts for 20 to 45 minutes, or until they turn the color of dark coffee with cream. If the nuts turn too dark, they can produce a sour flavor; if under-roasted the oils don't burn off and they aren't enjoyable.

Allow to cool, then use a nutcracker to open them. You can eat them now, or grind the nuts into flour, or smash them into smaller pieces to add to various recipes.

CALIFORNIA BAY NUT BRITTLE
A twist on the peanut-based classic.

Items needed:
Saucepan
Metal spoon
Candy thermometer
Cookie sheet
Parchment paper
Airtight container

Ingredients:
1 cup white sugar
1/4 cup water
1/4 cup maple syrup, or ½ cup light corn syrup
1 cup roasted bay nuts, coarsely chopped
1 to 2 tbsp. butter
¾ tsp. baking soda
¾ tsp. vanilla extract

First, combine the sugar and water in the saucepan. Turn the stove
to medium-low heat. Stir continuously until the sugar is completely
dissolved. Add your syrup of choice and continue to stir until it reaches
a low boil.

Attach your candy thermometer to the side of the saucepan,
ensuring its sensing end is submerged, but not touching the bottom of
the pan. Turn up the heat a bit and boil until the temperature reaches
250° F. Add the nuts, continue to stir, and bring to 300° F. This is known
as the "hard crack" stage in candy making.

Remove the pot from the heat and quickly add the butter, baking
soda, and vanilla, stirring until blended. The mixture will change in
texture at this point, and it might foam a little.

Pour the hot mixture onto a cookie sheet lined with parchment
paper. Using a large spoon or spatula, spread it out evenly. Allow to cool.

Once cooled, break the brittle into pieces and store in an airtight
container.

Linden

Tilia sp.

Family: Malvaceae
Parts used: leaf and flower
Medicinal actions: antispasmodic, de-mulcent, diaphoretic, hypotensive, nervine, sedative
Native geography: Europe, Japan; in North America, grows from Canada to Alabama, and west to Texas, Kansas, and North Dakota

My friend Saso said, "You've got to see this tree," as we drove through the Slovenian countryside. A countryside so picturesque I felt like I was driving through a fairytale with the mountains, waterfalls, lakes and idyllic little villages. I had never even heard of Slovenia but one day, just three months prior, the universe had decided it was a place I was destined to see.

I first met Saso in a San Francisco hostel early on in my medical training. Medical school can feel like one long, monotonous ride: eat, lecture, clinic, study, sleep. After a couple of years, you start to go a little stir crazy. I needed to see something other than the four walls of a lecture hall or my desk piled high with books. Being broke and only having a weekend I decided on San Francisco, a reasonable trip from Portland. Changing the scenery would give me new vitalization to push through the end of the term. And, I figured at the very least I could take stretch breaks by walking the pier, or up and down one of the mountainous streets of the city.

The first night I was doing my best to memorize the circulatory pathways of the body. The intricate pathways of connection that unite the entire human body in one big loop. The trouble was, I kept getting distracted by this one man sitting across the lounge from me. He was so animated and excited about whatever he was talking about that it made me irritated. My scholarly ego went into full blast, internally begging him to stop distracting me. It was a battle of my soul and my ego. My soul was desperate to know what his exaggerated hand gestures were

describing and my ego was trying to block everything out to study. What was I thinking? Hostels have no quiet, no privacy—they just aren't designed for study time. I decided to go to bed and to get up early. No one is ever up early at hostels, right?

At six o'clock the next morning, I made my way down to the kitchen. I had my plan all figured out. I would make a cup of tea and study for a bit before venturing out for a breakfast break. There was no one in the dining room and I heard nothing coming from the kitchen. Perfect. As I opened the kitchen door, I couldn't believe it: he was already there. He was hunched over the stove, watching an egg cook with serious determination. I saw him slice a tomato, put it and the egg on a piece of toast, and move to the otherwise-empty dining area. *Humph.* I stewed as I waited for my water to boil; I felt my insides starting to boil, too. A strange, conflicted feeling arose in my body and mind. Why was I so perturbed by this one human I'd never even spoken to?

I carried my tea into the wood-paneled dining area and sat several tables away. I watched the steam rise from my cup and dance in the morning light, streaming in through the window. All I wanted was peace, but for some reason I felt like a bee trapped indoors. My inside voice began screaming at me to make contact with this person, so I quietly got up and walked over to where he was sitting. I apologized for disturbing him and introduced myself. He asked me to sit down, and I noticed a patch on his jacket with a mountain, water and stars. "That," he said, "is the Slovenian flag." And that's how our friendship began.

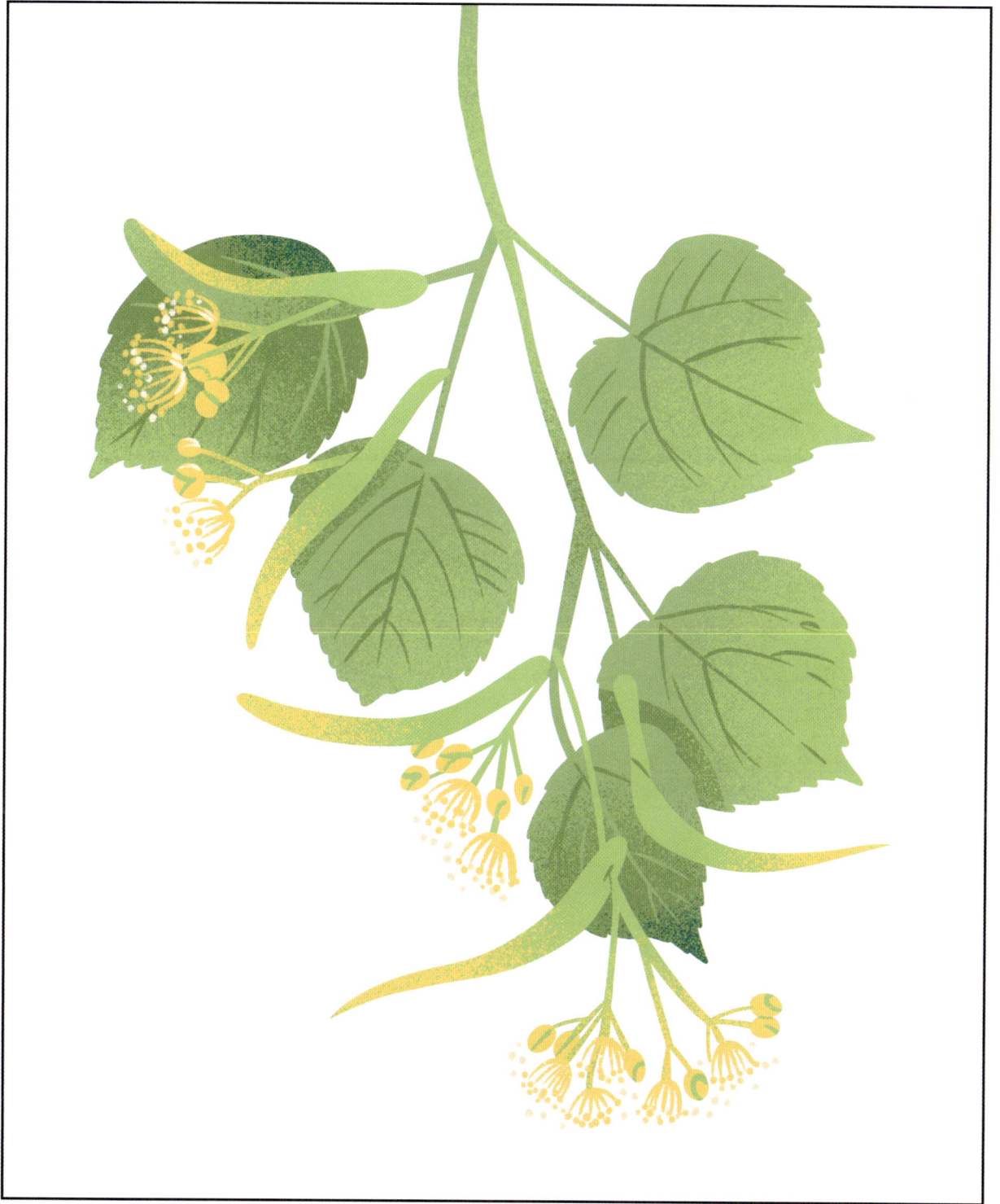

USDA hardiness zones: 3 to 8

Water: water regularly the first year; drought tolerant once established

Light requirement: full sun

Soil: moist, well-drained alkaline soil

Temperature: intolerant of frost

Wildlife notes: hosts small mammals and birds including cardinals, grosbeaks, wrens, woodpeckers, sparrows, thrushes, orioles, waxwings, nuthatches, and finches

Pollinator friendly: *Tilia cordata* produces mannose in its nectar, which may be slightly toxic to US native bees and wasps, who lack the enzyme to break it down. Choose a native variety if planting a new tree in North America.

Pests: linden aphid

As he told stories of Slovenia, I gradually realized why I had been so drawn to him—he spoke about his country with pride, and his eyes glistened as he described the beauty and magic that was deeply rooted in his culture. I never knew a country could hold nature as sacred as Slovenia apparently did. They had ancient stories about everything: their mountains, their animals, bells in churches, and even the countryside. There, oral history still weaves together culture and tradition. It was one of the first places I'd ever heard of that seemed to have its priorities straight. Music, poetry, art, literature, and liberty were infused throughout the tapestry of daily life. To an American, it seemed like a place of fairy tales.

Much later, as we drove through the Slovenian countryside with the Julian Alps as our backdrop, I marveled at the mountain peaks that went on for what seemed like forever. I'd lived in Colorado, but these mountains seemed to be on steroids. The closest common reference I can make is to the scenery in *The Sound of Music*. It's that majestic. Picturesque inns and quaint restaurants with the freshest food presented perfectly on a plate marked our journey. At the time, I had had very little European travel experience, but there was nothing about this place that felt pretentious or uninviting. Whenever we stopped to grab a bite or just to walk around, people would chat with us and ask where we were headed. "To Gogalova!" Saso would say. They'd all smile and say "Yes, yes, you must take her there!" I asked if we were going to see a tree, or if Gogalova was a different place. Apparently special Slovenian trees are given names, and Gogalova was the name of the linden tree we were headed toward.

"There!" he said. I followed Saso's pointing finger. Out in the middle of a beautiful field was the most picturesque linden tree I've ever seen. A giant trunk with wavy ridges supported a cloud of branches, leaves, and flowers that spread wide but somehow seemed to be growing in a perfectly symmetrical shape. It looked like something from a storybook. I envisioned us laying down a red-and-white checkered blanket under it, opening a wooden picnic basket, and laying out a simple feast of grapes, bread, and cheese. And wine. The scent of the linden flowers hung on the air, creating an intoxicating feeling of happiness mixed with pleasure. I was so overwhelmed I wasn't sure if I wanted to lie underneath it, stare at it in awe from across the field, or climb up into its branches to see what it sees from above. We did all three.

Saso told me how valued linden is in his culture. Some plant it for its summer shade or its fresh scent, but it was a tradition of the settlers to plant one wherever they built a home. It is a tree known for its longevity, so is associated with creating a blessing for the many generations to follow. When you are looking to symbolize a dynasty, choose a tree that will survive all the storms that come and go. A tree to remain the patron for the family for centuries to come.

The linden tree grows in a pyramidal shape in its youth; as it matures, it grows wide and round. The leaves are heart-shaped and have a fuzzy underside. The flower display begins in June and lasts for months. The flowers are white or creamy, with five petals that hang in clusters. They are very fragrant and highly attractive to pollinators. If you are in the US, please ensure you are planting a native species so as not to hurt the pollinator population. (See note at left.) Lindens are deciduous but aren't known for a fall display. They do offer a striking silhouette against a wintry background, however. With its perfect shape and stretching branches, it offers a nostalgic solace in the colder months.

Recently, I was sitting on my back deck when my daughter came out to chat. Of course I cherish the times we can just sit and connect. At one point, she asked me if she ever does anything that annoys me. Now, if you've got kids, you know this is a tricky question. But luckily I was of sound mind that day—I wasn't stressed or tired or in the middle of trying to accomplish 1,001 things. I reminded her that she is one of my absolutely favorite people in the world, and that the positive light she shines onto the rest of us is food for the soul. I asked her what made her ask such a question, and she was able to articulate the types of thoughts and feelings she often had at school. The uneasiness, the feeling that she'd done something wrong even when she'd done nothing wrong at all. At that moment, I realized she was beginning to experience true teenage anxiety. I made us two cups of linden flower tea. As the floral scent rose from the steam and the slightly sweet flavor graced our taste buds, she unfolded and released the torments of her troubled mind.

Anxiety can be described as a feeling of apprehension, tension, or uneasiness. A more severe type can lead to panic, the inability to breathe, dizziness, and heart palpitations. I don't need to research the statistics to know anxiety is becoming more and more prevalent within our society. The reasons why are part of our day-to-day and exposed through news outlets, social media, and inequalities.

Linden flowers are one of those subtle medicinals that work in powerful ways. I put them in the same category as chamomile. Delicate-looking flowers surprise us with their dynamo effect. I recommend linden to calm the mind any time anxious thoughts begin to percolate. It can be particularly helpful before bed, to inhibit the monkey mind that often clicks on when we lie down. Some say they feel a sedative effect after drinking it, so try it for yourself sometime when you don't have a long to-do list to determine how it affects you. On the flip side, I've prescribed it for stressed-out, overworked executives; such people often seem to be able to drink it all day long with no onset of fatigue. My conclusion is that for people with high cortisol levels, there will be no sleepiness effect but rather an ability to help focus thoughts in high-pressure environments. Linden's natural sweetness also makes it a great syrup that is safe for kids. I use it with my young son if his "on" switch (aka he is super hyper) can't seem to turn off.

Linden is a great addition when fighting a cold, as it helps to clear the nasal passageways and respiratory tract of excess mucous. And with the flu, give linden if there is profuse sweating with no resolution of fever, or when shivering is present with alternating chill and fever. If there is fever with excessive sweating yet the fever doesn't break, beware of dehydration and give linden tea frequently, even in tablespoon-size doses.

Linden Recipes

_____

INDICATIONS

- Anxiety
- Colds
- Fever
- Flu
- Heart palpitations
- Hyperactivity
- Indigestion
- Insomnia
- Nervous headaches
- Nervous vomiting
- Nervousness
- Panic attacks
- Restlessness

*Generally regarded as safe for all populations. Fatigue might be exacerbated in those with fatigue syndromes. Consult with your health care practitioner before use if diagnosed with heart disease.

LINDEN FLOWER SYRUP

When the sweet floral aroma of the linden blossom arrives, I know it is time to take full advantage of all this tree has to offer. Try this syrup on pancakes, in mocktails and cocktails, added to tea, or in any recipe that calls for a hint of honey-like sweetener.

Collect linden flowers just as they open, preferably in the morning hours when the dew is still present. The flowers are surrounded by a bract, which is the long, green leafy-looking element. I find it easier to take my pruning shears and trim the whole blossoming piece initially, then once I'm back in the kitchen I'll use my shears to remove the flowers from the bract. You could compost the bract, but you can also dry it and add it to the leaves for tea.

Items needed:
Pruning shears
Saucepan
16-oz. glass mason jar
Storage bottle for finished syrup
Fine-mesh strainer

Ingredients:
1 cup water
1 cup organic cane sugar
¼ cup lemon juice, freshly squeezed
1½ cups fresh linden flowers

Place the water, sugar, and lemon juice in the saucepan. Slowly bring to a boil while stirring, and continue stirring until sugar is dissolved. Turn off the heat and let it cool slightly. You want it to still be warm when you pour it into the mason jar.

Put the linden flowers into the mason jar, and pour the boiled liquid over them, ensuring they are fully submerged. Give a stir and close tightly. Put the jar in the refrigerator or store in a cool, dark place for 2 to 3 days. Be sure to shake or stir it daily.

Strain the syrup with a fine-mesh strainer. Be sure to squeeze every last drop from the linden flowers, then pour the syrup into storage bottles until you are ready to use it. Linden syrup will keep in the refrigerator for up to 6 months.

ANTI-COLD, ANTI-STRESS AND
ANTI-INFLAMMATORY TEA

Linden is one of those herbs that is highly beneficial to keep on hand. Kids love it, and because of its sweetness, it is easy to blend with other spices and herbs to customize to your needs.

Items needed:
Saucepan or teapot
Tea mug

Ingredients:
2 to 3 cups water
½ cup linden flowers and leaves
1 cinnamon stick
2 to 3 dried apple slices
1 to 2 cloves
¼ cup rose hips
Tiny pinch of ground ginger

Put all ingredients in the saucepan and bring to a boil. Turn the heat to simmer, cover the pot with a lid, and let it simmer for 3 to 5 minutes. Turn off the heat, but leave the pot covered and let the tea steep for 10 minutes.
    Strain, then enjoy.

London Plane Tree

Platanus x acerifolia

Family: Platanaceae
Parts used: bark, seeds
Medicinal actions:
analgesic, anti-inflam-
matory, antimicrobial,
vulnerary
Native geography:
southeastern Europe,
United Kingdom; now
common in many cities
along the US's eastern
seaboard

When I first visited New York City, it wasn't the skyscrapers or the lights of Times Square that caught my attention, but a certain prevalent street tree with sprawling branches and camouflage-looking trunks. They were everywhere my daughter and I walked, these giant trees. They looked to me like creatures from a childhood story, creatures with twenty outstretched arms of varying lengths, twisted and bent in every direction. When I went to touch the bark, I found it cool and smooth, despite the patchwork of white, olive green, cream, and gray. Some of the larger trees were shedding their bark in long strips. You could pull on a corner and it'd come off in one long strip, from bottom to top.

I had been dreaming of adding a new location for my herb shop, in New York City. Like many people, I had a sort of fascination with New York, and held that naive belief that New York only consisted of New York City. As a kid, it's the only part of the state that I ever heard about—it was the land of Patti Smith and the Chelsea Hotel and Led Zeppelin concerts. I'll admit I got starry-eyed whenever someone mentioned the place.

I had opened my first herbal apothecary, The Herb Shoppe, in Portland, Oregon, while in graduate school. People thought I was crazy to try for a second location so far away. I always replied with the plain fact that some of my classmates were having babies; this would be my baby, but easier since I got to close and lock the door at seven p.m. I didn't have a Daddy Warbucks to back me, but I had a dream I believed in and I knew how to work

hard. I leveraged my student loans, ate a lot of ramen noodles, and opened my doors in September 2005. It was the glorious good ol' days before social media or e-commerce. I used an old red leather, felt-lined jewelry box as my cash register.

A few years after opening, we experienced two major events. The election of Barack Obama as our 44th president, and a major recession. Emotions fluctuated between joy and despair. As people struggled to make ends meet, lost jobs and health insurance, my shop became a bridge to healing. We never turned anyone away. It was during this time that I began to realize that my community herb shop was more than just a retail business struggling to make money; it was a safe place, one where people could ask for real help. Herb shops are gathering places where people feel moments of peace, places where people listen when you talk. I began to dream bigger and wondered whether all this newfangled technology would let me open a second location in a place where health care options were sorely needed. As I let the idea simmer over time, I continued building my Portland shop, but ideas and inspiration for that expansion kept popping up.

I had a flash of inspiration on April 19, 2011. Anyone who knows me well can tell you that Led Zeppelin is my all-time favorite band. Despite missing their heyday, I had seen Robert Plant play during his Now and Zen tour when I was fifteen, and *Led Zeppelin III* is literally how I survived high school. On this particular day, I hadn't even had a chance to shower before dropping off my ten-month-old

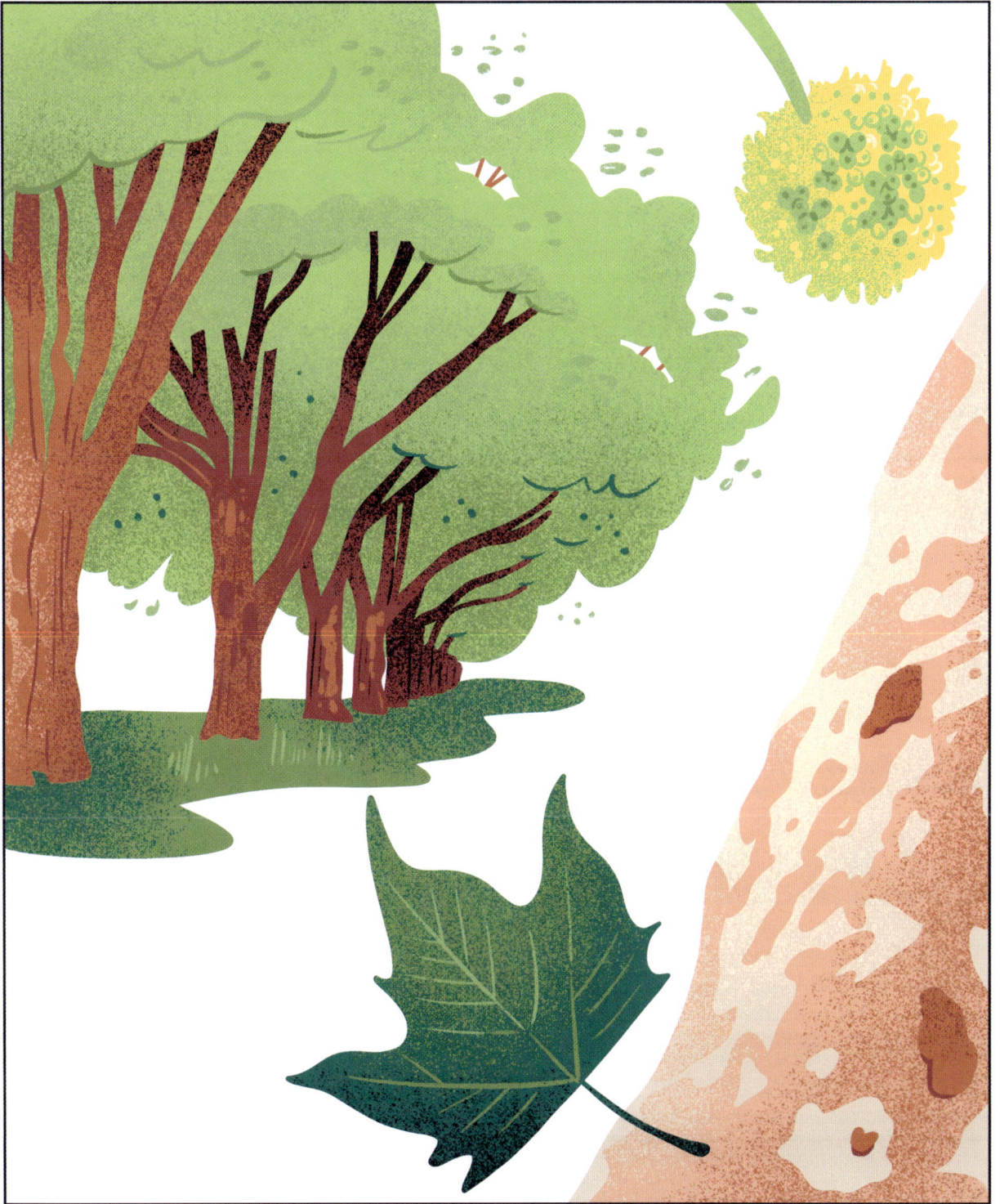

PLANT DATA

USDA hardiness zones: 5 to 9

Water: keep the soil moist to a depth of 18 to 24 inches

Light requirement: Appreciate full sun but tolerate part shade

Soil: average, medium to wet, well-drained soils

Temperature: cold tolerant to -20°F; also tolerant of hot summers

Wildlife notes: the seeds are eaten by squirrels, muskrats, and beavers; hummingbirds eat the dripping sap

Pollinator friendly: wind-pollinated; the female flowers form a spiky fruit that blows away; over the winter, its outer coat breaks down and releases the seeds

Pests: sycamore anthracnose, and canker stain

at daycare and then rushing to the shop to see patients. As I put acupuncture needles into my last patient at the end of the day, I felt relieved to have a few moments to rest while the needles did their work. As I stepped out of the treatment room and into the main shop, I felt pleased that it had been a busy-but-productive day, but in my state of hunger and fatigue I almost didn't recognize the man standing in line in front of me, waiting patiently to be helped. It was the one and only Robert Plant. My heart nearly pounded out of my chest, but I sauntered over calmly and asked him if there was something I could help him find. "Mint tea," he said. My hero, my savior, simply wanted some regular, plain mint tea. He mentioned that he liked to drink it on stage while performing. I fumbled over my words and gushed, at times inappropriately, but we managed to have a relatively lively conversation. After we wrapped up, I walked him out— and to the bus stop. *Robert Plant* rode the bus back to his hotel downtown. I sat down on the bench to catch my breath. I saw him make his way toward the back of the bus, and noticed that he chose to stand instead of sit down. He had on a red cotton scarf with little tassels—I'd always known he had flair. I was certain the day had been a sign from above.

Five months later, I opened The Herb Shoppe, Brooklyn. All it took to push my dream into a reality was one conversation with another dreamer. And now I walk the streets of New York looking at these magnificent London plane trees while listening to "Whole Lotta Love" by Led Zeppelin, which was recorded at London's Olympic Studios but mixed in New York, in case you didn't know.

There are so many reasons to plant a London plane tree. City planners love them because they are a fast-growing tree capable of filling large spaces quickly. The seeds are incredibly quick at germination, too, taking only a few hours to sprout on their first day in the sun. The London plane has proven to be resilient in almost any growing condition including in compacted soil, in drought, in high heat and in air pollution. The leaves and the bark work like mini air filters, binding pollutants in exchange for off-gassing cleaner oxygen. One London plane tree reduces atmospheric CO_2 levels by 5 pounds. The shade canopy can provide reprieve from any hot summer day or cover from the rain. In the spring, male and female flowers both appear on the same tree; the male flowers are yellowish while the female flowers show a red/purple blush. The female flowers turn into cute little cylindrical balls that appear in pairs. They are dense with seeds on the inside, and the fuzzy-yet-stiff spikes on their exterior help with wind pollination.

People are often concerned when they see the bark shedding from the trunk, but this is normal. Exfoliation is a yearly event, mainly due to the tree growing so rapidly it can't keep up with its own trunk expansion unless it replaces bark at a rapid rate. But it also helps reduce the toxic burden of the accumulated pollutants, pests, moss, or other negative exposures. Think of it like a big, hairy dog who's just come out of the lake—you know it's going to shake.

The London plane is actually a hybrid tree. Creating a hybrid is easier than it may sound. You can accomplish this by cross-breeding, or by grafting two plants of the same species. Cross-breeding is done in three steps and is typically recommended for flowering plants:

1. Using the male part of one plant's flower (the stamen) to pollinate the female part of a different plant's flower (the pistil);
2. Harvesting the fruit that the pollinated flower produces
3. Growing the seed.

In the seventeenth century, someone decided to cross-breed the American sycamore with the Oriental plane. Voilà, the London plane.

Let's look at each species individually, and then at the combined genetics of the hybrid to better understand how to use it medicinally. Oriental plane leaves have been used (and researched on mice) for their ability to reduce both pain and gastric ulcer inflammation. *The Canon of Medicine* (1025), a five-book compendium, was compiled by a Muslim and Persian physician-philosopher, Avicenna. He recommends Oriental plane for any type of inflammation-related pain, such as toothache or knee pain. While it's still used today as a tea, research has shown that a tincture of Oriental plane produces the strongest medicinal effect.

When we review the medicinal actions of the American sycamore, we see similar actions of use. Cherokees used it for digestive upset, pain, diarrhea, and to wash wounds of the skin. In fact, the Native American Ethnobotany database gives great examples of how a tribe may have used one plant in various ways, to treat many different things. Many plant medicines can be used this way, changing the medicinal action based on how it is prepared.

With hybridization, you never know exactly which traits will come through, but the London plane has been proven to treat conditions of the urinary system, stomach, digestive tract, and skin well into modern times. It is another great example of using whatever resources are close by. When I was working at my herb shoppe in Brooklyn and my little girl cut her arm on a random jungle gym bolt, I didn't have the backyard medicine variety I was used to in Portland. But a quick assessment showed me the abundance of the city. I collected, washed, and applied slightly bruised London plane leaves over her arm. She slept pain free, and by morning the wound was well on its way to healing.

London Plane Tree Recipes

INDICATIONS

- Bladder complaints
- Burns
- Conjunctivitis
- Diarrhea
- Ulcers
- Wound healing

BLADDER BLISS TEA

A nourishing tea for the bladder and urogenital system. Drinking tea is one of the best ways to support our body's waterworks system overall. Since tea is ingested internally, the healing elements come into direct contact with the kidneys and bladder. The beautiful seeds of the London plane tree make a strong cup of tea and act as an ally to this entire system.

Items needed:
Quart mason jar

Ingredients:
1 tbsp. London plane tree seeds
½ tbsp. corn silk
½ tbsp. uva ursi
1 tbsp. dried chamomile
1 tbsp. dried lemon balm

Put all the ingredients into the mason jar, then pour almost-boiling water over them, filling it to the top. Close the lid and let it steep for 4 hours. Strain.

Drink three cups per day. You can drink it at room temperature, reheat it, or drink it cold. The colder you drink any tea, the more diuretic its effect.

TOE AND TOOTH RELIEF VINEGAR

My husband seems to stub his toe a lot—*a lot* a lot. I don't really under-stand it, because the table or chair that is the culprit of such violent attacks is often one that hasn't moved in decades. Yet somehow, his brain and his toe seem to forget their place in space on a regular basis. I always say that toe and tooth pain are the two worst types. Though small in terms of area, when either is in crisis it can really ruin our day.

Items needed:
Saucepan and lid
Fine-mesh strainer

Ingredients:
1 oz. London plane tree bark
4 cups apple cider vinegar
5 drops clove essential oil

Add the apple cider vinegar to the pan and bring it to a low boil. Add the plane tree bark and cover with a lid, leaving it slightly ajar. Be sure the heat is low and simmer slowly, until the liquid is reduced by ⅔.

Strain with a fine-mesh strainer and put the vinegar mix into a dropper bottle.

Add the clove oil, close the bottle, and give it a gentle shake.

When needed, apply it on a cotton ball and place the cotton directly onto the toe or tooth. You can also use a cotton swab for a smaller, more direct application.

Magnolia

Magnolia grandiflora,
Magnolia x soulangiana,
Magnolia officinalis

Family: Magnoliaceae
Parts used: bark, flower
Medicinal actions:
aromatic, astringent,
bitter, diaphoretic,
digestive, febrifuge,
stimulant, tonic
Native geography:
China seems to be the
consensus but perhaps
other parts of Asia and
North America. Today
they are indigenous only
to Southern China and
the Southern United
States. Eight species of
magnolia are native to
the United States.

I got my own bedroom when I was six years old. My parents decided to put an addition on our house, which meant I could transition into their old bedroom, my sister would take my brother's room, and my brother would move into the basement. He originally was going to move into the attic, but had seen a ghost on the attic stairs one day and decided the basement was a better idea. My sister was more excited about all these changes than I was. I liked sharing a room. I think little kids innately find it comforting. It makes the night less scary and provides a lot of opportunity to talk about things not spoken of during the day. Our room's walls were a bright sky blue, a color that made you think of *Sesame Street* and swimming pools. A giant mirror stretched the length of an entire wall. Underneath the mirror, on opposite ends, were matching built-in dressers and little desks. They were varnished with layers and layers of the shiny orange so popular in the 1970s and early 1980s. The only other thing I remember being in the room was a rug, our record player, and the bunk beds.

Despite her regular displays of annoyance, I was grateful I had my sister with me when I went to sleep. She would tell me funny stories to help me drift off. When I really needed it, she'd stretch her arm down from the top bunk just so I could touch it in the dark and confirm that she was still there. Sometimes we'd pretend her arm was a bridge from her "island" to mine. She would bop her head against her pillow in a consistent rhythm for me, which gently shook the bunk bed frame. The vibration lulled me to sleep.

My mom worked very hard to get my new room just right. We went to the wallpaper store and leafed through huge catalogs that were heavy and thick in order to find a pattern that I would want to look at each and every day. I chose tulip clusters that were painted in the primary colors of red, blue, and yellow on a white background. The carpet store was next, and we landed on bright grass green—so I could pretend I was laying outside and looking up at my new flowers, you see.

Once I moved into my new room, I had to develop a fire escape plan (tie sheets together and lower myself from the second story), get used to sleeping alone (my stuffed animal collection suddenly grew), and adjust to the change in light. Formerly, my room was on the back side of the house; now I was in the front, overlooking the yard. Our saucer magnolia tree was right outside my bedroom window. This tree had an amazing display. It was the superstar of our yard. Sure, as a kid I thought it was pretty when it bloomed, but I only truly appreciated it for practicing my tree-climbing skills. I did notice how everyone else in our family—and even pedestrians who walked by—would comment on how pretty it was. So one day, I decided it must be something special and that I'd better start paying attention to find out what all the hubbub was about.

That spring, when the soft wooly buds formed, I plucked them from the tree and rubbed them against my cheek. Their softness reminded me of the fake fur on my bunny rabbit–shaped piggy bank. Over the coming weeks, I watched those buds suddenly unfurl into perfectly imperfect flowers. The flowers

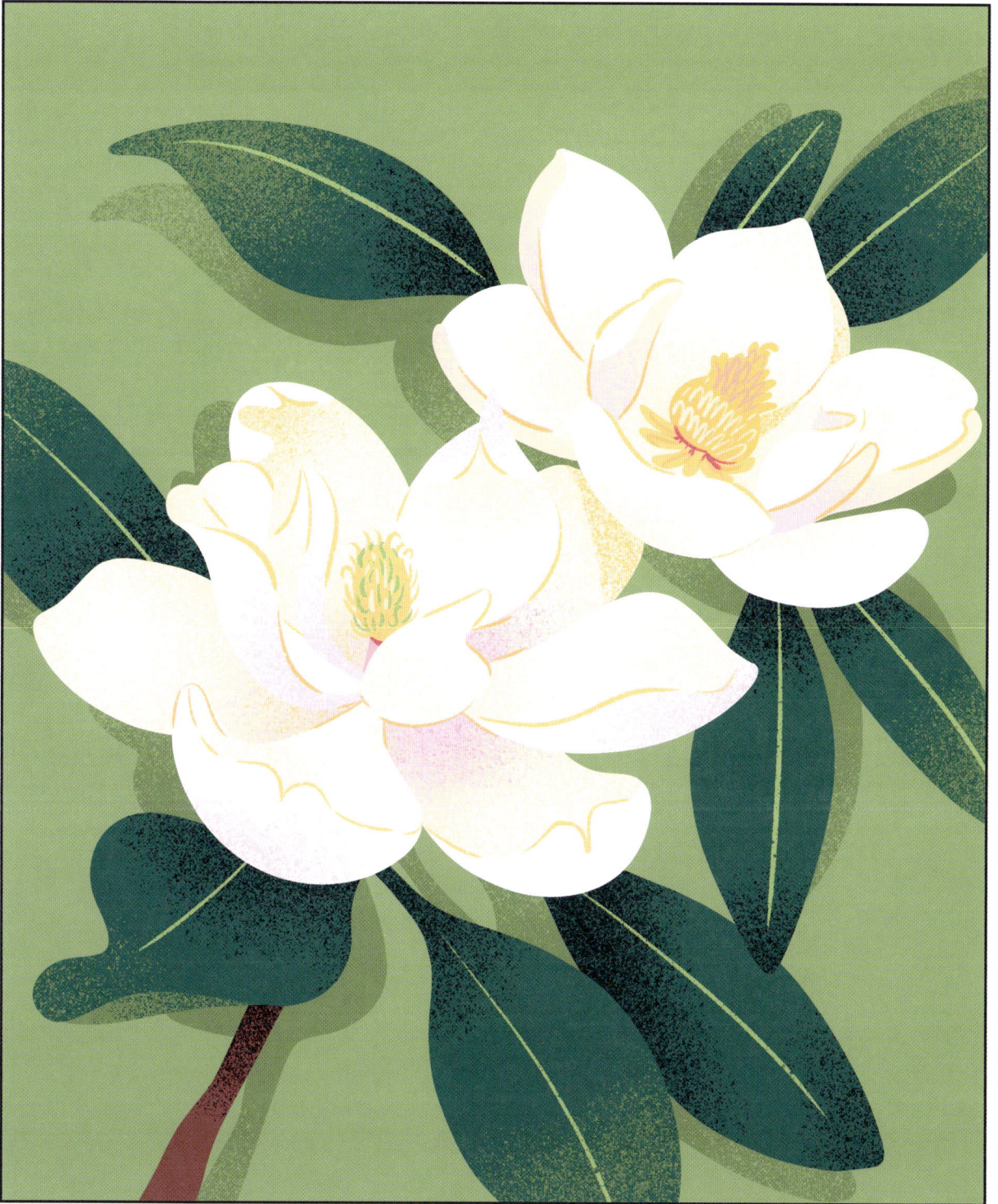

USDA hardiness zones: 3 to 9; the hardiness of different varieties can vary

Water: mulch helps shallow roots to improve drainage and water absorption. Water twice a week for the first six months of the seedling's life.

Light requirement: full sun

Soil: well-drained; root rot occurs if tree sits in water

Temperature: requires protection below 20° F

Wildlife notes: beloved by songbirds, woodpeckers, cardinals, and finches

Pollinator friendly: bees, wasps, ants, and flies all feed on magnolia; in some parts of the world, magnolias provide year-round nourishment

Pests: magnolia scale, verticillium wilt, algal leaf spot, canker, aphids

were a combination of blue, pink, and white all rolled into one. Their scent would waft through the neighborhood, announcing the blooms' presence to everyone. I'd never paid attention to that transformation before. It made me think of the show we watched every Sunday, *Mutual of Omaha's Wild Kingdom*. Sometimes they showed time-lapse videos, and observing this in real time made me feel a bit like the host of the show, Marlin Perkins.

With that tree just outside my window on the second floor, I felt like my room was almost an extension of the tree. I began to watch it closely from season to season. At the end of winter, I'd anxiously await the arrival of protruding buds, which would then miraculously produce a woolly fur—I thought of it like a winter coat protecting the delicate flowers inside. Many days I would pull up a chair and just watch out the window as birds came by to land on its branches and to see the squirrels play chase up and down its trunk. After a couple of years, I could tell when the flowers were about to pop open by the scent the tree produced as a precursor to blooming. I would close my door each morning on my way out to school, leaving the windows cracked just in case that day was the day the flowers released their petally fragrance. I knew if they opened while I was at school, the aroma would have filled my room. For weeks as its flowery display beckoned every neighbor for blocks, I'd hide away in my bedroom lying on my carpet of green, appreciating the tulips on the wall. As the exclamations from the sidewalk drifted up to my ears, I would smile and think, "Yes, I agree, it is an amazing tree."

During my training as an acupuncturist, we delved deep into the study of Chinese herbs. Magnolia is just one of hundreds of plants in Chinese medicine that have been safely used for thousands of years. As an acupuncturist (and naturopath), we look at the patient as a whole versus focusing on treating individual symptoms. We are assessing qi, the energy of the body and of each organ, to determine if it is healthy and balanced. We are also evaluating the fluids of the body—generally termed "blood" in Chinese medicine theory. Are they moving throughout the body as they should? Is there a blockage of flow, or perhaps is there too much flow or too little? I observe and question new patients thoroughly to get a broad sense of why they have come and then I use the diagnostic tools of feeling the pulses and looking at the tongue to discern further information. When the patient is anxious or there is chronic stress, the pulse will often feel wiry and the tip of the tongue will be red and have prickle dots. This is when I consider using magnolia.

Despite researchers finding over 250 different constituents in magnolia, the primary focus has fallen to two specific ones; honokiol and magnolol. These constituents are powerful antioxidants that scavenge up the free radicals in our body that can damage cells and often cause cellular malfunction. The more free radicals you have, the faster your skin ages and the higher chance you have of chronic diseases of the heart, liver, lungs, and intestines developing. It has been shown that honokiol and magnolol are over 1000 times more potent than vitamin E, which is often taken as a supplement specifically to combat free radicals and reduce inflammation. These two compounds are also known to benefit asthma sufferers and the digestive tract, and to ameliorate fat accumulation, insulin resistance, and adipose inflammation.

But magnolia has a specific affinity for calming the central nervous system to reduce stress, lessen anxiety, and reduce insomnia. In one study, honokiol was found to be five times more effective than the commonly prescribed prescription drug Valium, without the side effects. Magnolia also activates the cannabinoid receptors, the same relaxation-promoting receptors as cannabis. This is particularly helpful to aid in falling asleep.

I don't see how you could go wrong by planting a magnolia tree in your yard. The big, ovate, deep green, and glossy leaves were a favorite of mine to collect as a child—a bunch strung together instantly created a natural fan for a hot day or pretend play. Adults seem to be more interested in the decadent blooms and their scent. Tight buds are often protected by a fuzzy fur on the cap—I encourage you to run your fingers over them, acknowledging the promise of the bloom to come. Magnolias are long-lived, and one can be appreciated by many generations. magnolia tree planted by Andrew Jackson at the White House in 1828 lived to be 190 years old. Plan space for it accordingly, to allow it to live out its full life cycle.

Magnolia Recipes

INDICATIONS

- Abdominal bloating
- Anxiety
- Asthma
- Belching
- Cancer
- Diabetes
- Diarrhea
- IBS
- Skin, anti-aging
- Stomachaches
- Stress
- Vomiting

CHOCOLATE-DIPPED MAGNOLIA BLOSSOMS

Let me count the ways we can turn a beautiful magnolia blossom into a delectable treat. While they're as much treat as medicine, I promise that these chocolate-covered blossoms will taste like nothing you've had before.

Items needed:
Double boiler
Tongs
Cookie sheet
Parchment paper

Ingredients:
12 magnolia blossoms, still closed but close to opening
2 cups couverture chocolate; either dark or milk so long as it has a high cocoa and fat content, which helps with smooth melting and dipping
¼ cup organic cane sugar

Gently wash the blossoms in cold water and pat dry.

Set up your double boiler and begin to melt the chocolate. Keep a close eye on it, stirring often to ensure it doesn't get scorched on the bottom of the pan.

Line your cookie sheet with parchment paper.

Sprinkle the blossoms with sugar. Then, using the tongs, gently dip them into the melted chocolate. Usually one dip is enough, but sometimes I'll let the first dip harden slightly and then give it a second dip.

Once dipped, lay each blossom on the lined cookie sheet. When you've dipped all 12 blossoms, place the cookie sheet in the freezer to chill for at least 4 hours.

You can eat them as-is, but if you're going to serve them, they are best served on a chilled plate. Another option is to use them as decoration on top of ice cream.

MAGNOLIA STRESS-RELIEF SYRUP

A teaspoon of this syrup is helpful to reduce stress and give your central nervous system a little bit of support.

Items needed:
Saucepan
Stirring spoon
Fine-mesh strainer
Bottle for storage

Ingredients:
2 tbsp. magnolia petals
1 tbsp. dried passion flower
½ tbsp. oatstraw
⅛ tsp. ground ginger
2 cups water
1 cup organic sugar

Put 2 cups of water into a saucepan and bring to a boil. Add all the herbs, turn off the heat, cover, and let steep for 30 minutes.

Strain out the herbs by pouring the liquid in the saucepan through a fine-mesh strainer, then return the liquid to the saucepan. Bring to a low boil and add the sugar. Boil, uncovered, until the liquid is reduced by half. Turn off heat and allow to cool before pouring into a storage bottle.

Maple

Acer sp.

Family: Aceraceae
Parts used: bark,
leaf, sap
Medicinal actions:
antispasmodic,
astringent, expectorant,
galactagogue
Native geography:
most species originated
in Asia, but nine species
are also considered
native to North America,
eleven to Europe and
Western Asia

"Things grow here that don't grow any-where else in the world." This is what a forest woman told me once when I was living in Bellingham, Washington. You might be wondering what a "forest woman" is; the best way I can explain it is a woman who was born, raised, and still lives near the forest. This one in particular was speaking of the scenic mountain ridge of the Chuckanuts—a ridge that's part of the Cascade mountain range but is also its own unique landmass where moun-tain and sea meet. The ridgeline is only about twenty-two miles long, and it bends ever so slightly to encompass a crescent-shaped bay. The word itself, Chuckanut, originates from the Nooksack tongue and translates as "a long beach far from a narrow entrance."

When I moved to Bellingham, I didn't have a car, but quickly realized I was going to need one if I was ever going to get to Chuckanut. I'd heard about a guy with a Volvo graveyard who sold cars for cheap. I was the perfect candidate for a station wagon or boxy 1990s sedan. After working double shifts for a bit, I scraped together $500 and paid him a visit on a rainy day. I scanned the dismal landscape—dilapidated Volvos of all sorts everywhere I turned. They ranged from com-pletely destroyed to what seemed moderately decent? After a long walk around and looking at flat tires, peeling paint, and misshapen bumpers, I set my sights on a white classic 1980 sedan. The owner, who had been creep-ing along next to me the whole time in his little Bobcat, seemed pleased I'd finally made up my mind. He drove it over to the front of my new car and, after attaching a chain to the

front bumper, pulled a few levers and began lifting it out of the sticky mud. Witnessing all of this happening, I seriously re-contemplated my decision, but then I quickly put on my blinders and squealed about how cute it was!

He quickly hosed it down, and as I watched the mud slowly dripping down and off the car, he scrounged around for some keys. He got in to try and start it as I held my breath and crossed my fingers. But I kid you not—the thing roared right to life on the first try. My intuition had confirmed my belief that only a Volvo could instantly start after sitting outside for months. I hopped in, turned on the radio (joyfully noting that it had a cassette player), and drove home. Now that I had a set of wheels, I had my sights set on exploring the wilderness around me: Index Town, Baker Wilderness, Wing Lake, Tipso, Picture Lake, and Nooksack Falls were all on my list. But I decided on visiting Chuckanut first. This town where I'd ended up was like a nature lover's wonderland. Having grown up landlocked with my only view never-ending flatlands, I felt like a pioneer. Bellingham had a scenic byway, and I was ready to spend an entire day driving down the Chuckanuts to Samish Bay.

My plan was to drive to Larrabee State Park, then hike up to Fragrance Lake—ending what would be a hot trip at an alpine lake sounded both refreshing and magical. I hit the trail with exuberance and, like a Labrador, it was hard to focus on any one thing because there was so much to look at. The flora and fauna were thick and growing from every direction, which made me feel like I was in prehistoric times. It all seemed so untouched

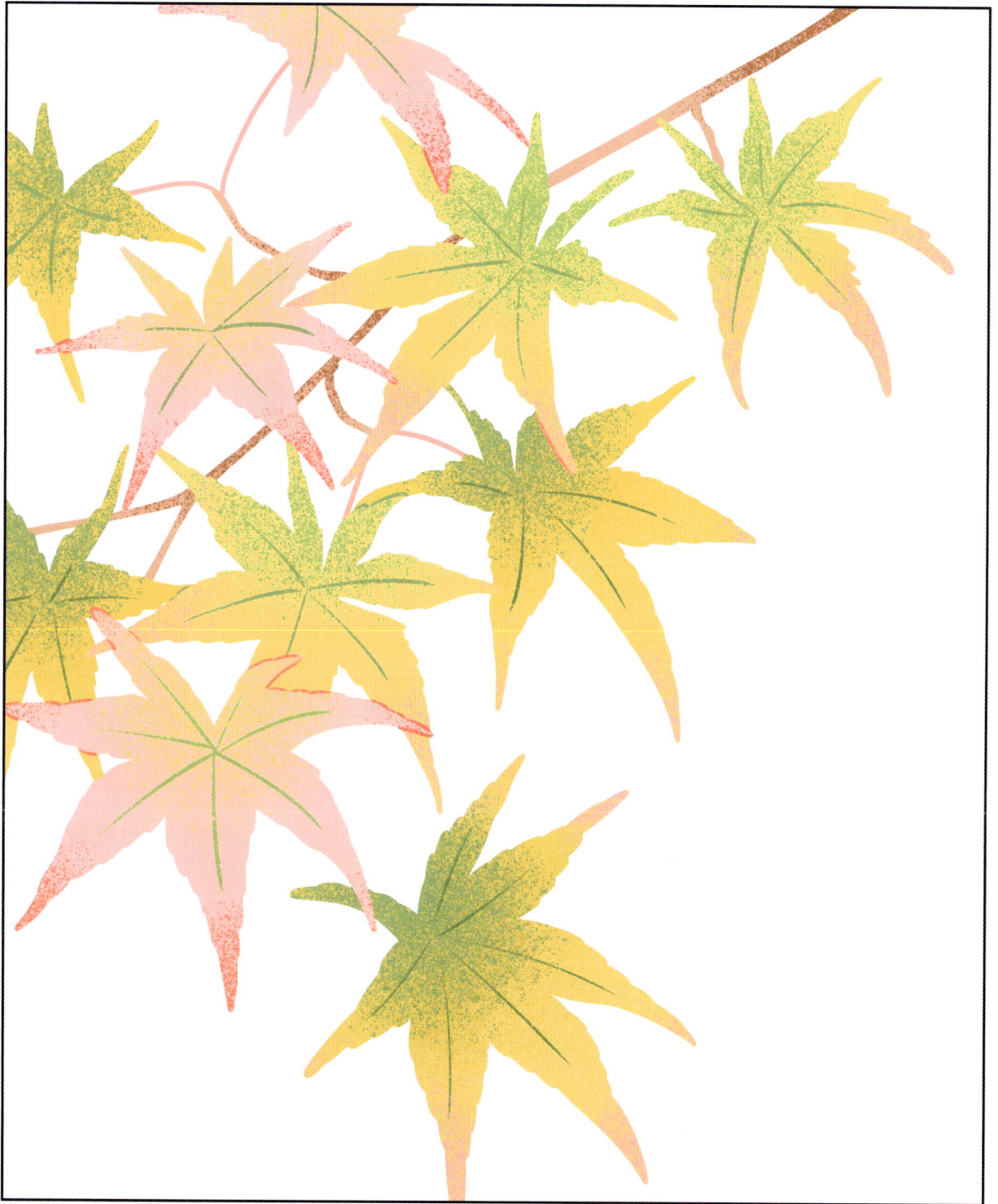

USDA hardiness
zones: 5 to 9, with
some species hardy
to zones 3 and 4
Water: mature maples
need about one inch of
water per week; they
grow faster in moist
conditions
Light requirement:
full sun to partial shade
Soil: moist, well-drained,
acidic soil
Temperature: varies by
species; most Acer are
hardy to -10°F
Wildlife notes: squirrels
and chipmunks store the
seeds and the cavities in
the red maples species
along rivers attract
ducks and other ground
nesters
Pollinator friendly:
valuable to honey bees,
bumble bees, hover-
flies, flies, and beetles;
some species are only
wind-pollinated
Pests: anthracnose,
fungal leaf spots
(including tar spot),
powdery mildew, and
verticillium wilt

by human existence. At age twenty-six, I would often embark on hikes without doing much research in advance, and within a quarter of a mile I found myself on a steady uphill climb. It seemed to last forever. I suddenly understood what the guidebooks really meant by "elevation gain." My breathing became more labored with each step. I may as well have been climbing flights of stairs or on that horrible stair machine at the gym. Because I was looking down a lot to watch my footing, I noticed a leaf on the trail—a leaf bigger than my entire head. If I'd seen a bigleaf maple before, I must have been distracted because I was instantly shocked by its size. It was not perfectly symmetrical, but it was perfect in every other way, with a strong and sturdy, short stem. I paused and held it up to the dappled sun to inspect its bright and glossy deep green color. I contemplated the incredible design the bigleaf maple's foliage as I put one foot in front of the other—up, up, up. I was so busy twirling the leaf with my fingers I didn't even notice that I'd reached a plateau. An ever-expanding view of Samish Bay started to unfold before me, and in the distance I could see the San Juan Islands. A view where the sky meets the sea and misty hills rise up through the scattered clouds. I could have stayed right there all day.

But curiosity pushed me onward, toward my goal. The trail flattened out and birds and more plants kept me company. At one point a dog that looked like a white wolf strode onto the trail in front of me. It completely surprised me; no human in sight. We paused and examined each other for a minute before he bounded back into the woods. Through tunnels formed by arching branches above and more bigleaf maples, I wove my way deeper into the woods until suddenly, as if by magic, Fragrance Lake appeared. I felt like I was standing in an Old Master oil painting—a

small lake completely surrounded by a forest, twinkling in the glow of afternoon light. Growing up I used to call this particular slant of light "the yellow light." It always appears around four o'clock in fall. The sun hits the horizon just right, and you feel like you are immersed in and surrounded by that yellow warmth of light. Here, though, it was still summer. A haze hung over the water, and gnats floated lazily on the air above it. I half-expected some mythical goddess to rise up out of it. Then it hit me: I could be the goddess. I stripped down, dove into the water, and became part of the picture.

———————

I grew up knowing that maple was helpful for many of the day-to-day complaints that cropped up at home. I watched my grandma make an eyewash for her cataracts with it, and also use that same brew for the hives we kids got when we ran through the woods. The bark makes a great gargle for sore throats and helps ease the gripping pains of indigestion and menstruation. Many different Asian populations have used red maple for centuries to prevent cardiovascular and cerebrovascular diseases.

Modern research has validated the ways in which my elders used maple. But more so, they have discovered even more uses. Forty species and eleven subspecies of Acer have demonstrated a broad spectrum of medicinal actions. Recently, it was discovered that its prebiotic properties target chronic inflam-mation and support the metabolic system by aiding the growth of healthy bacteria like lactobacillus and bifidobacillus. When we improve the gut, the body can devote more to fighting infection and inflammation. After noticing Acer's astringent action on the gut lining and its ability to modulate short-chain fatty acid production, researchers began to study its effect on elastin and collagen. Turns out that maple leaf extract inhibits the breakdown of elastin and maintains the complex reinforcements of collagen. A specific constituent of red maple leaves, glucitol-core containing gallotannin (GCG), has shown promise in the fight against obesity and insulin resistance. It is proposed the GCGs accomplish this by modulating butyrate- and acetate-producing bacteria. These bacteria balance gut microbiota and maintain the mucosal barrier. In turn this supports the immune cells in the lining of the gut, which prevents infections.

Studies also show maple's affinity for the liver and supporting hepatocytes (liver cells). This action gives the liver a hand up when combating any disease by ensuring the healthy cells stay healthy.

Acer also inhibits photoreceptor cell death. One study with mice demonstrated that Acer prevented retinal degeneration by modulating protein expression and preventing the thickening of the outer retina layer.

I have twelve maples on my property. I recently planted eight "flame" maples after living for ten years with my other four, which just don't change color in the fall. Honestly, with all the amazing maple species out there, why in the world would you plant ones that don't offer a fall display? In Oregon, people look very forward to fall maple displays. Afterward, the deciduous leaves drop. They begin to leaf out again in early spring, usually April. It seems to happen all of a sudden. Waiting for buds to emerge is much like watching the kettle boil; the moment I turn my back, boom, they're all leafed out. An interesting fact is that bee colonies decide whether they are going to swarm in the spring approximately six to eight weeks before the bloom—with their sensors so in tune with nature, they can determine if their current hive is too small for the upcoming year. If so, you'll see them swarm in spring.

Maple Recipes

————

INDICATIONS

- Cataracts
- Coughs
- Digestive complaints
- Heart tonic
- Hives
- Immune tonic
- Inflammation
- Insect bites
- Lactation
- Skin health, anti-aging
- Sore throat

MAPLE LEAF MOMIJI

Momiji means "maple" in Japanese; this recipe is for fried maple leaves, a traditional snack in Japan. My kids go crazy for them.

Note: This is a plan-ahead recipe; you need to preserve the leaves in salt for weeks beforehand.

Preservation:
Items needed:
Plastic storage tub, approximately 7.5 quarts

Ingredients:
Freshly picked Japanese, red, sugar, or silver maple leaves
Salt

Harvest your maple leaves in the summer, when they are fresh and vibrant. Wait until midday to gather them so that the morning dew has evaporated. Collect them directly from the tree, not the ground.

Next, dry the leaves for about 24 hours. I tie a sheet around the backs of four chairs and lay the leaves on top. This allows for air to circulate above and below, making for even drying.

In your clean storage tub, spread a layer of fine salt on the bottom, then lay down your first layer of maple leaves. Continue creating alternating layers of salt and maple leaves until you've used all your leaves, ending with a layer of salt on top. Close up the container tight and store in a cool, dark place for one to nine months.

Frying:
At this point, you can decide to fry the maple leaves with or without batter. If frying without batter, just drop them into safflower oil in a frying pan, and they'll quickly fry up. Remove, lay on a paper-towel-lined plate to drain. Cool, then eat.

Items needed for batter version:
Mixing bowl
Frying pan
Plate
Paper towels

Ingredients:
1 cup flour
1 cup milk
1 egg
Enough safflower oil to fill a frying pan 1 inch deep

In the mixing bowl, combine the flour, milk, and egg. Whisk until smooth.

Add the oil to the frying pan and turn the heat to medium.

When the oil is hot, begin dipping the leaves into the batter by their stems. Lay them out flat in the frying pan, unfurling their leaves if necessary so that they retain the maple leaf shape.

Fry them on each side 1–3 minutes, depending on batter thickness and oil temperature.

Once done, place them on a plate lined with a paper towel to drain and cool.

Season them however you wish. Try a seasoned salt or nutritional yeast, or perhaps pour maple syrup on top or frost with a little icing.

Noni

Morinda citrifolia

Family: Rubiaceae
Parts used: fruit,
leaves, seeds
Medicinal actions:
anti-inflammatory,
antioxidant, astringent,
carminative, demulcent,
tonic
Native geography:
Pacific islands, spe-
cifically Indonesia to
Australia; it is now naturalized in tropical areas
spanning a wide swath
from South America to
India and Australia

No one had mentioned the howler monkeys. I lay in bed, listening to them throughout the night, my unaccustomed ear terrified of the noises I was hearing. Their loud, whooping roars sounded sinister in the darkness. Add to that sensation the smell of fresh noni fruit decaying on the ground all around my tree hut—my senses were simply overwhelmed in the unfamiliar environment of Belize. How such a beneficial medicine could stink so bad was beyond me. I prayed I wouldn't have to get up to use the bathroom and have to navigate any of it.

When I stepped off the plane in Belize City, I wasn't sure what to expect. I had studied with my teacher, Rosita Arvigo, for years, but never at her home. The air was moist and thick, and my skin sucked up every drop. I could see palm trees just outside the airstrip. I looked around for my ride—as has happened on many of my adventures, I wasn't exactly sure who I was supposed to be meeting. After a few minutes of ignoring the taxi drivers who were repeatedly approaching, I noticed a passenger van parked near a group of white people standing around. "That looks about right," I said to myself. I made my way over.

I was there to learn about mental health from the Mayan perspective, and to expand my herbalism training. Herbalism is often a very straightforward learning experience: here is a plant, this is what it does. But sometimes, the study of the plant's spirit can offer more insight than any book, and a good teacher with experience can teach you a plant's highest healing potential. Just like people, plants are unique and individual and can offer healing gifts for both physical and nonphysical ailments. My job for the next week was to listen, assimilate, and get curious about how a culture so different from my own treats physical and mental health.

This newly formed group of strangers headed toward the Macal River and the nature preserve Rosita lived on. She had magically secured land and a house on the outlying perimeter, her home eternally encroached upon by jungle vines and plants wanting to swallow up anything that didn't belong. The casita sat on a bluff with a giant flat terrace off the main room. You could see the horizon line no matter which direction you turned, which made it difficult to identify any single cardinal direction. The view was extensive: endless treetop canopies, birds in flight, flowers bursting forth on giant vines as they snaked their way up tree trunks, and gentle mists that would rise up at night only to fall back down with the rising sun.

My abode for the week was a short walk from Rosita's house, along a trail through the jungle where we could observe the plants, chat among ourselves, or walk in meditation. I instantly knew the noni was close by when I got a whiff of the familiar scent of something like decaying vomit. Sure enough, not too long afterward, I stepped on one rotting on the ground. I had initially had a love-hate relationship with noni, simply because of the smell. But over time, I've grown to love it. The fresh juice vitalizes me in a unique way that can be hard to describe—but for anyone over the age of forty, know that it makes you feel like you are twenty again.

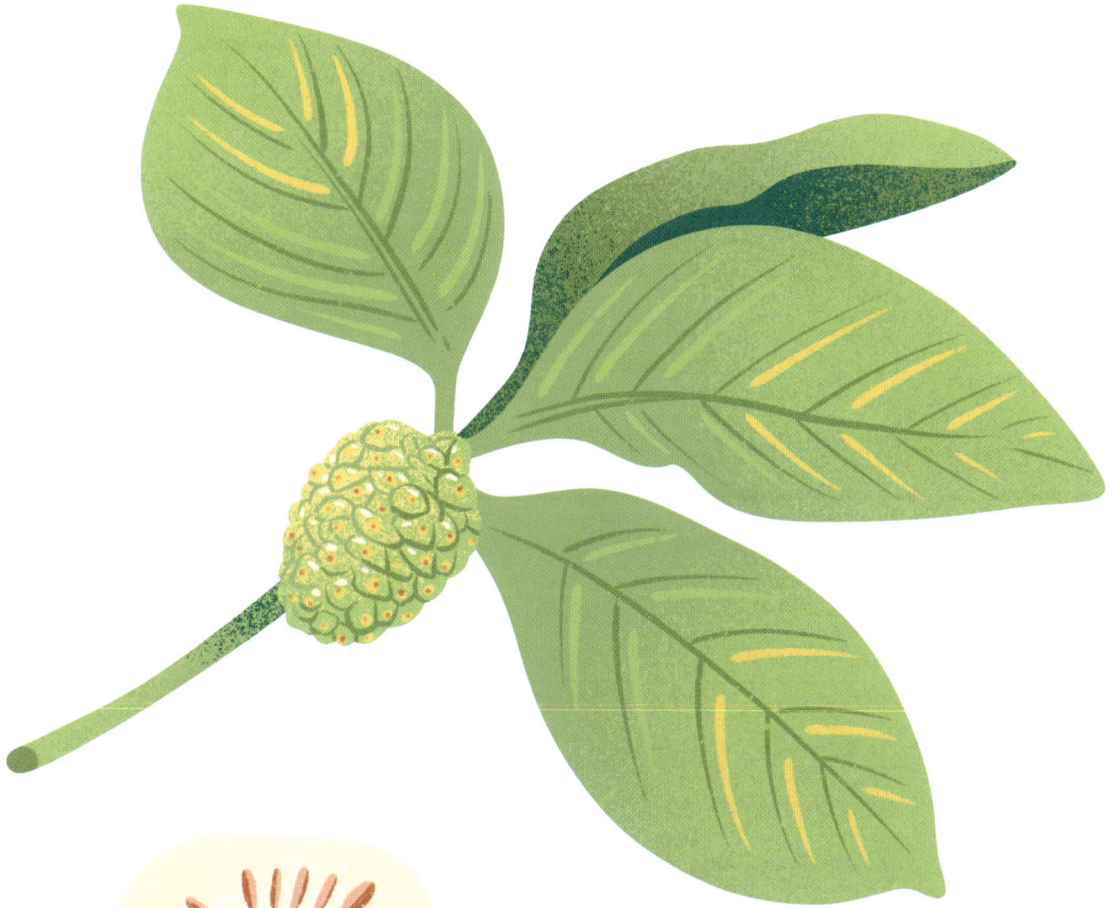

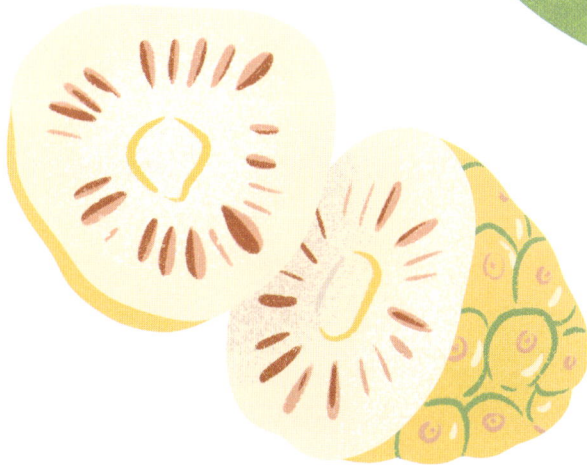

USDA hardiness
zones: 10 to 12 outdoors, and 4 to 11 indoors
Water: water deeply the first 2 to 3 years after planting
Light requirement: Full sun
Soil: well-drained; a cinder-soil mix works well
Temperature: intolerant of frost
Wildlife notes: bats, birds, small mammals, and cows eat noni fruit
Pollinator friendly: bees love the flowers, and it has been hypothesized that some of the medicinal qualities noni retains come from bees
Pests: aphids, scales, spider mites, weevils

I unloaded my backpack in my one-room cabana on stilts. There were two beds, but I'd been given a room to myself because they didn't know what gender "JJ" was from my registration. We had been advised to check the room for scorpions each night, as they tended to sneak in and hunker down to stay safe from predators. Immediately, my overactive imagination created a mental picture where I was trying to hunt for scorpions in the dark—there was no electricity—by bending down to look under the bed with my flashlight. Panic started to set in when I realized I wouldn't know what to do if I actually found one.

For a week, I learned Mayan culture and the origins of what they believed caused most diseases. A few examples: susto (fright or trauma), pesar (grief and loss), tristeza (sadness, depression), coraje (anger), mal ojo (evil eye), and invidia (envy). The treatment for these conditions was what they call a "spiritual bath." This is a custom-blended bath soak of plants, flowers, bark, or leaves, that matches healing properties specific to the patient's suffering. Creating one is a sacred task, from gathering the plants to macerating them by hand in water and singing healing prayers along the way. After the mixture steeps in the sun, it's added to a bath in a ceremonial way to release a patient's trauma, suffering, and pain.

And afterward, the patient rests. We silently wrap them in a blanket and gently lay them down to recover, contemplate, or sleep. We sweep and wash away the remains of the petals, leaves, and bark that have given their all to the healing process. Often, we offer a glass of noni juice too, which we make by mashing it over and over with a wooden pestle. We push and squeeze every last drop through a strainer and pour it into a cold glass, offering its nectar to the patient as the first taste of a new life.

Noni is an acquired taste. When I first drank noni juice, I was told to not smell

it beforehand, just to shoot it down. Can you guess what I did? Smelled it of course, and instantly regretted it. This incredibly unique-looking fruit produces a healing juice that lights up your insides, but it smells horrible. The scent lands somewhere between spoiled fruit, rancid cheese, and vomit. It's something special for sure. But back to the first time I drank it: I was in Puerto Viejo in Costa Rica, a tiny town on the country's southeastern coast. As many young travelers do, I was flying by the seat of my pants with plans and ended up staying a bit out of town, right on the beach. I noticed an older man who lived next door collecting the noni fruit. Being the ever-curious herbalist, I walked over and asked him how he planned to use it.

As I sat on an old tree stump, I watched him make me a fresh glass of noni juice. He told me he drank it every day, for his eyes. He had started to get cataracts but swore that the noni was keeping them at bay. "It is the old person's medicine against aging," he said with a chuckle as he handed me the glass. I had a big drink. Luckily, it does not taste anything like it smells. What I noticed, almost immediately, was clarity of sight. It was like everything I saw became sharper, crisper, and more vivid. The instant effect took me by surprise, and I remained in a state of wonder the rest of the day.

———————

I've come to use noni for many different things, and prefer, if possible, to use it fresh. Think of it as a daily tonic to supercharge the body against all the daily challenges we encounter: stress, pollutants, inflammation. I was taught that the noni fruit is ready once it's dropped from the tree but before it begins to spoil. This allows the fruit to ferment a bit, which enhances its medicinal properties. Once soft, you can just cut it up and throw it into the blender with a bit of water. The leaves and seeds have their own medicinal uses, but in the juice they provide healthy fiber.

The fruit and/or just the leaves, made into a tea, can be ingested for gout. Gout, which is caused by uric acid building up in the joints, and particularly smaller joints like toes, can be extremely painful. Uric acid is produced when there is an excess of xanthine oxidase (XO) in the body, which makes uric acid. The more XOs, the more potential for gout. Noni is good at stamping out XOs, reducing and/or preventing gout. You can also dab a tea made with the leaves topically for ringworm, a very common but pesky skin infection.

Because noni was hyped up commercially in the early 2000s, there have been quite a few studies performed about its benefits. Research papers on noni point to its ability to prevent cancer, lower high blood pressure, fight infections, reduce rates of diabetes, and improve athletic performance. All can be found via a quick search on Pubmed or on the National Institutes of Health website.

Most people won't want a noni tree or shrub in their yard because of the mess the fruit makes after it drops, but if you have an affliction it can treat, it is worth considering. This fruit-bearing tree is in the coffee family. Once mature, it will continuously produce fruit. The fruit starts off bright green, turns to white, and resembles a small pineapple or lumpy potato. Five-petaled, white, star-shaped flowers open on the fruit, a few at a time. They have a sweet, musky scent. The fruit itself does not smell so good, particularly when it falls from the tree and rots.

Noni Recipes

INDICATIONS

- Arthritis
- Burns
- Cataracts
- Diminishing vision
- Diabetes
- Fatigue
- Gout
- High blood pressure
- Infections
- Parasites
- Ringworm

Generally regarded as safe for all populations. Those with any type of kidney disease should use caution. Noni is high in potassium and may interact with blood pressure medications.

NONI MUFFINS

These delicious muffins are a great way to incorporate noni fruit into your weekly routine.

Items needed:
Stand or hand mixer
12-cup muffin tin

Ingredients:
1 cup organic cane sugar
¾ cup vegetable oil
2 large eggs
½ cup mashed noni
1 cup shredded carrots
½ cup mashed overripe banana
2 tsp. vanilla extract
2 cups flour
2 tsp. baking soda
2 tsp. ground cinnamon
¼ tsp. salt
½ cup chopped walnuts

Beat together oil and sugar with the mixer. With it running on low, add in the eggs, noni, carrots, banana, and vanilla until smooth.

Add the flour, baking soda, cinnamon, and salt.
By hand, stir in the walnuts.
Scoop the batter into the muffin tins.
Bake at 325° F for 35 to 45 minutes.

NONI FRUIT LEATHER

The perfect snack on the go—and much healthier than
store-bought brands.

Items needed:
Blender
Dutch oven
Dehydrator and silicone sheet pan liners (trust me, this makes it so
much easier!)

Ingredients:
1 pound washed, ripe noni fruit
1 tsp. pectin
1 tsp. calcium water
1 cup organic cane sugar or white grape juice concentrate

First, puree the noni fruit in the blender. Add it to your Dutch oven and
set the pan on the stove.

Add the calcium water to the puree. Turn the heat on medium-low.
If you are using sugar, add it now, stirring until dissolved and the puree
starts to simmer.

If you are adding grape juice concentrate, put it in the blender and
turn it on. Add the pectin with the blender running to emulsify the two
together; this usually takes a couple of minutes. Then add this mix to
the noni puree and stir for one minute.

Next, ladle out the puree onto your silicone-lined dehydrator trays.
Keep in mind that this should be a very thin layer, thick enough to
make a roll-up, but not too thick that it will take forever to dry. Finding
this perfect thickness takes practice, so don't get discouraged if it isn't
perfect the first time.

Dehydrate on low, 110° F, for 12 to 14 hours, depending on your
climate and the thickness of the puree.

Once dried, cut the leather into strips and roll them up. Store in an
airtight container at room temperature, or in the refrigerator.

*Note: I've run out of space, but definitely look up how to make noni goat
cheese as well. It's easier than you think—and delicious!*

Oak

Quercus alba,
Quercus robur

Family: Fagaceae
Parts used: inner
bark of smaller
branches and twigs
Medicinal actions:
astringent, tonic
Native geography:
Quercus alba exists
in eastern and central
North America from
Minnesota to Ontario,
Quebec, and southern
Maine to as far south
as northern Florida and
eastern Texas; *Quercus
robur* is native to most of
Europe and western Asia

A corns were my treasure when I was little. I would obsessively collect them, coveting each and every one, believing them to be as individual as snowflakes. I kept them in an old metal *Star Wars* lunchbox that I'd converted into my personal treasure chest. They would rattle and roll inside as I walked around the neighborhood, making a special kind of music just for me. Most of the thousands I gathered had fallen from giant oak trees that belonged to my neighbor, Mrs. Catherine Weaver—Mrs. Weaver to me, since as a product of the '70s I would never have dreamed of calling an adult by her first name.

Have you ever started collecting something and found it difficult to stop? Maybe you were picking berries, or searching for the perfect pumpkin at the pumpkin patch? That is how collecting acorns was for me. It was so difficult to stop—each one was so perfect. The cupule, the little cap that sits on the top of the nut, reminded me of a hat. And while collecting them was my primary pursuit, feeling the crack-split-crunch of a dry nut under my shoe also gave me a distinct satisfaction. The trees themselves also provided incredible canopies of shade that provided immediate reprieve from the hot, dense, Midwestern summer air.

I immediately sensed that Mrs. Weaver was unique when we moved in next door. The first time I caught a glimpse of her was through her big bay window. The double curtains were usually drawn, but sometimes the heavy set would be pulled back and you could see the sheer lavender inner set, slightly blowing in the draft from a vent that must have been close by. I was doing what kids did back then and exploring everything outside—including Mrs. Weaver's yard— when one day, there she was, standing just behind those lavender curtains, trying to catch a glimpse of me. Her posture made her seem tall, but in reality she was only 5 feet. Her hair was short, dark, and permed into little tight curls. Her eyes sat behind dark cat eye glasses. As one of the lavender sheers suddenly got pulled to the side, a shiver went down my spine. I was thinking I was about to get yelled at for being in her yard, for one thing, but also so curious about those purple curtains. Our house's décor embraced its era, and was all orange shag carpet and fake wood paneling. I'd never seen such delicate exoticness, and my inner princess persona was instantly enthralled. Being a child who completely lacked any sense of subtlety, and who desperately wanted to meet the woman who owned those lavender curtains, I started to wave vigorously.

And that's how a friendship that has now spanned over fifty years started. The first time I went into her house I don't think I was actually invited, but my unbridled four-year-old spirit compelled me to walk right past her and into the room I had to see. Not only were the curtains purple—so was the couch, the carpet, and even the wallpaper. It was glorious. I imagined her laying on the chaise longue in the afternoon watching Merv Griffin or Dinah Shore and sipping iced tea. But this was just one of the magnificent rooms she had to show me. There was a waterbed in her oldest daughter's room—a bed made of water?! My

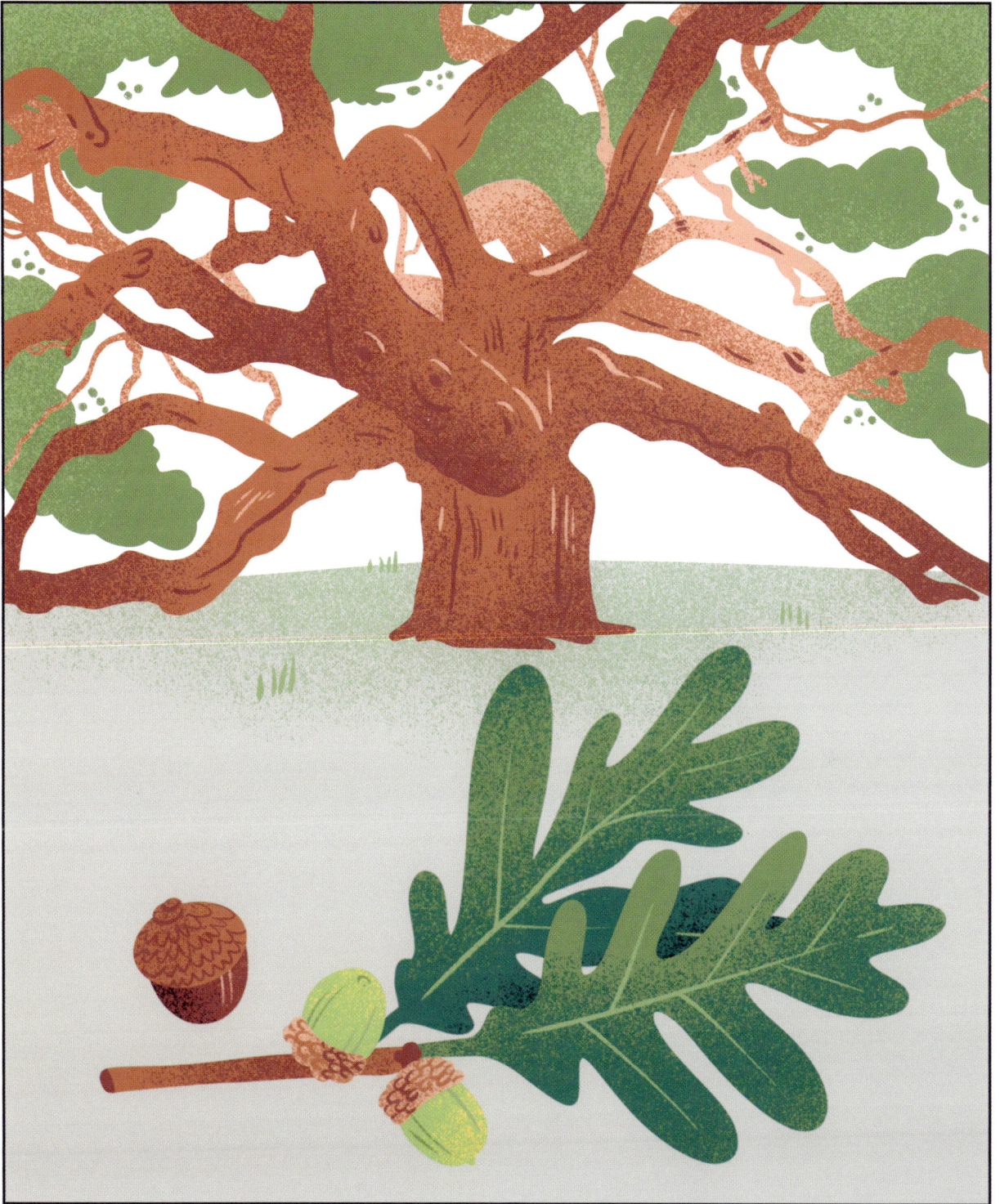

USDA hardiness zones: 4 to 9

Water: deep root system makes oaks drought tolerant once established

Light requirement: sun, part shade, even forest understory

Soil: deep, moist, rich, slightly acidic soil

Temperature: one of the most resistant trees to damage from ice and snow

Wildlife notes: owls like to nest in white oaks, but many birds and mammals utilize its resources

Pollinator friendly: attracts butterflies and supports hundreds of species of caterpillars

Pests: white oaks are the most resistant to disease and insects of any oak species

mind was blown wide open. Out the back door was a deck that wasn't your regular square or rectangle shape. Oh no, this spectacular woman had an octagonal-shaped deck, complete with a flowing fountain. I remember the feeling of fascination as I watched the water recirculate over and over, its gurgling lulling me into another dimension.

But it was the kitchen that I would grow to love as if it was my own. Wildly bright and filled to the brim with knickknacks, various salt and pepper shaker sets, and modern items like a spice rack, handheld whisk, and toasted sandwich maker. At home we had boring white Corningware plates with that cornflower stamped in the middle. At Mrs. Weaver's, even snacks were eaten off fancy floral plates of varying sizes. Over the years, I'd spend countless hours at the vinyl-covered kitchen table while she'd do whatever task needed to be completed, all the while chatting away and never acting like I was a bother. She talked to me like I was a real person, somehow always knew what I was feeling, and shared with me objects and experiences outside of my own world.

Once we became besties, I regularly showed up unannounced, ready to explore her glamorous and fascinating world. She had a cactus garden I loved to visit in particular because one, I'd never seen a cactus, and two, no one had a cactus garden in Nebraska. I knew they grew in foreign places I'd never been to, like California and Arizona. The knowledge that Mrs. Weaver had traveled to those places made her even more exciting to me. I would also say hello to each and every frog statue on her deck—there were at least twenty—as I'd run in through the back door. Sometimes we would examine leaves and acorns together, and it was from her that I learned you could make flour and then bread from the acorns.

These days, I watch my own kids collect acorns. We'll lay them across the back deck and think of 1001 different ways we could use them. When we get tired, we scoop them all back up and add them to our treasure chest/lunchbox, which sits by a ceramic frog in our own cactus garden.

———————

There is something special about having an oak tree nearby. Perhaps it is because of the way they intertwine with our own long cultural heritage, since they play a major role in several belief systems from around the world. Or because they feature as characters in countless pieces of fiction. Or since they produce one of the most easily identifiable leaves in the world. And say what you will about the mess acorns can cause—many wildlife species depend on storing them for winter survival. You can even collect acorns for yourself and mill them into acorn flour to turn into bread.

There are also few better astringents than white oak. With its high tannin content, white oak pulls tissues together in a way that drains fluid accumulation and puckers in the remaining healthy cells. It is a reliable medicinal with consistent results and blends well into formulas as a supporting herb. I often recommend it for hemorrhoids, the irritating swollen veins around the rectum that can cause pain, itching, and/or bleeding. A number of different things can cause them: gut inflammation, food intolerances/sensitivities, pregnancy, straining during bowel movements, even stress. Sometimes, when the inflammation calms down, they will retract on their own. But many times you need to apply a strong astringent to pull the vein back up and into its correct position. Using white oak both internally and externally often aids in a speedy recovery and rehabilitation of this delicate area. To take it internally, drink a medicinal-strength tea three times a day, or take a tincture. To treat the area externally, I recommend a sitz bath.

On the border of Herefordshire and Worcestershire in the United Kingdom lie the Malvern Hills. The area is famous for its natural mineral springs and wells, and a healing spa was opened there in the early nineteenth century. It was said that the waters were so pure that they aided in all health and healing processes. One technique used at the spa was the sitz bath. The term "sitz" comes from the German verb sitzen, which simply means "to sit." Beautiful stone chairs were constructed with a bowl as the seat so that the patient could lie back but have their hips, abdomen, and pelvis submerged in the water. They were used to treat issues with digestion, menstruation, vaginal problems, and the lower rectum. I frequently recommend sitz baths and yes, sometimes patients look at me like I'm crazy. So much work, they say. But when you target a problem with specific tools to treat it, it often resolves quickly and efficiently. While we don't have those incredible Victorian-era sitz bath chairs around now, we do have Dollar Store plastic tubs, which are often perfectly sufficient to do the job. Remember, targeting the area is the goal, which is why we don't just take a bath, which would dilute the treatment. Begin by setting the plastic tub inside a bathtub. Fill it up with medicinal-strength brew, which can be warm, room temperature, or cool. Once your desired temperature is reached, lower your bum into the plastic tub and bend your legs out in front so they rest in the larger bathtub. The idea is to get as much of your abdomen and pelvis into the plastic tub as possible. Bring a good book with you and sit there for 15 to 20 minutes.

Oak Recipes

INDICATIONS

- Bladder tonic
- Cough
- Diarrhea
- Goiter
- Gum, mouth, and teeth tonic
- Hemorrhoids
- High blood pressure
- Lack of appetite
- Prolapse: bladder, intestinal
- Puffy eyes
- Runny nose
- Sinus congestion
- Skin eruptions
- Thrush

Generally regarded as safe for all populations. Some speculation has arisen regarding safety for those with cardiovascular, kidney, and liver disease. Avoid during pregnancy.

BUM BUM SITZ BATH

Oak is one of the best herbs for healing sensitive tissues and pulling them back together when inflammation or injury has occurred. Combine that aspect with a topical application, via a sitz bath, and you get instant relief from pain and swelling from hemorrhoids, childbirth, fissures, and lower pelvic pain.

Items needed:
Large pot
Strainer
Plastic basin big enough for your rear end to fit in. Ideally it will be deep enough to reach your belly button when you're sitting in it as well. I've seen commercial sitz baths advertised recently, but they act more like a bidet and I find them too small. Something like a large dishwashing tub works great.

Ingredients:
12 cups water
2 oz. oak bark
½ oz. butcher's broom
½ oz. echinacea root

Bring water up to a boil and add all the herbs. Simmer on low, covered, for 15 minutes. Strain out herbal elements.

Allow the herbal-infused water to cool until it is bath water temperature. Pour it into your sitz bath. Submerge your bum and pelvis, keeping any extra brew close by to refill as needed. Sit in the tub for 15 to 20 minutes.

OAK ICE CREAM

This recipe is so unique and too good not to share. Makes 1 quart.

Items needed:
Ice cream maker
Saucepan
Strainer
Stand or hand mixer

Ingredients:
3 cups whole milk, macadamia milk, or hemp milk
  (use a high-fat milk here)
1¼ cups heavy cream or high-fat non-dairy creamer
1 cup medium-toasted oak bark
12 tbsp. organic cane or turbinado sugar
4 tbsp. honey
1 tsp. salt
8 large egg yolks

First, prep the ice cream maker; most of them require that you freeze an inner chamber for some time before use.

In your saucepan, bring your milk, creamer, and oak bark to a boil. Reduce the heat to keep it at a low boil, and maintain a simmer for 8 to 10 minutes while stirring often. Then turn off the heat, cover, and let it steep for 1 hour.

Strain the oak bark from the liquid, then return the liquid to the saucepan. Turn the heat to low.

With a stand or hand mixer, whip the sugar, honey, salt, and eggs for approximately 2 to 3 minutes, until the ingredients have doubled in size and look very fluffy. Stir in ⅓ cup of the oak infusion from the saucepan to temper the mixture. Blend well.

Take the sugar mixture and add it to the oak infusion in the saucepan. Stir gently but thoroughly until well combined.

Next, cool the ice cream base down by setting it into an ice bath, but be sure to stir from time to time to promote even cooling.

Transfer to the ice cream maker, following manufacturer's directions. Freeze for 1 hour before eating.

Pine

Pinus sylvestris

Family: Pinaceae
Parts used: bark, pollen
Medicinal actions:
analgesic, anodyne,
antibacterial, appetite
suppressant, aromatic,
depurative, stimulant
Native geography:
Pinus sylvestris is the
most widely distributed
pine in the world; it can
grow from mountaintops
at 8000 feet all the way
down to sea level. Most
of northern Europe and
Asia have native popu-
lations; it's now widely
distributed across the
United States.

G liding up a ski lift under falling snow is one of my favorite feelings in the world. Even though you are moving, it feels like time has stopped. The deafening quiet presses pause on daily concerns as you steadily fly over snow-laden pine tree branches bending with nature's weight: snow. To be higher than the pines is a special feeling. How often do you get to see the top of a pine tree? We are always looking up at them from underneath, but on a ski lift, you get the rare glimpse of what a bird, perched on the top, gets to see.

I grew up in Nebraska, a place known for Cornhusker football, women's volleyball, our giant water aquifer, corn, and tornadoes. It's a place where you don't have to drive far to get to the country. Once you are there, you can literally lie on your back and see the curvature of the earth because there is so much sky and the topography is so flat. Fireflies and light-ning illuminate summer nights, and heading to the basement when weather warning sirens go off is commonplace. It's a perfectly nice place, but for a tree person, there is one thing lacking: pine trees. While some varieties, such as the ponderosa pine, can be found in little clusters clinging to existence in our extremely hot, dry summers, they are rare. We need to head over to our neighbor, Colorado, to really see pines.

Colorado was our playground. We shared a man-made border, but I was repeatedly amazed at the stark difference between Nebraska's forever-flat terrain and Colorado's peaks, valleys, and plateaus. How could two states be so close together, and yet worlds apart? I often wondered why in the heck we'd moved to Nebraska if Colorado had been an option! But luckily, my dad liked to take road trips, and he was all about seeing the nature Colorado had to offer.

In the '80s, ski fashion was hitting an all-time peak and heading to the mountains to ski was definitely the thing to do in the winter. Despite lousy weather conditions, we often drove nine hours in snow, sleet, and ice just to experience a fun family ski vacation. We'd all be stressed out by the time we arrived from having slid off the road or watching my dad white-knuckle the steering wheel while trying to see the road through a blizzard. My mom did her best at trying to keep everyone calm, using the sing-song voice moms sometimes do when they are acting like everything is normal. I recently drove my own kids up to Mount Hood Meadows in winter here in Oregon, and as I gripped the wheel, I won-dered how in the hell—or maybe a better ques-tion is, *why* in the hell—had my parents put three kids in a station wagon with no seat belts to slip and slide their way through mountain ranges? All I could come up with was that they were determined to make memories—just like I was trying to do.

Our first-ever trip to Colorado was to Vail. And as we left the plains of Nebraska, rows and rows of pine trees started to completely cover mountainsides. I had never felt so small as we drove on carved-out roads along steep valley walls between high mountain peaks. My dad, perhaps the least "cool" dad in the world, seemed to think himself a connoisseur of all worldly things: wine, foreign food, the stock

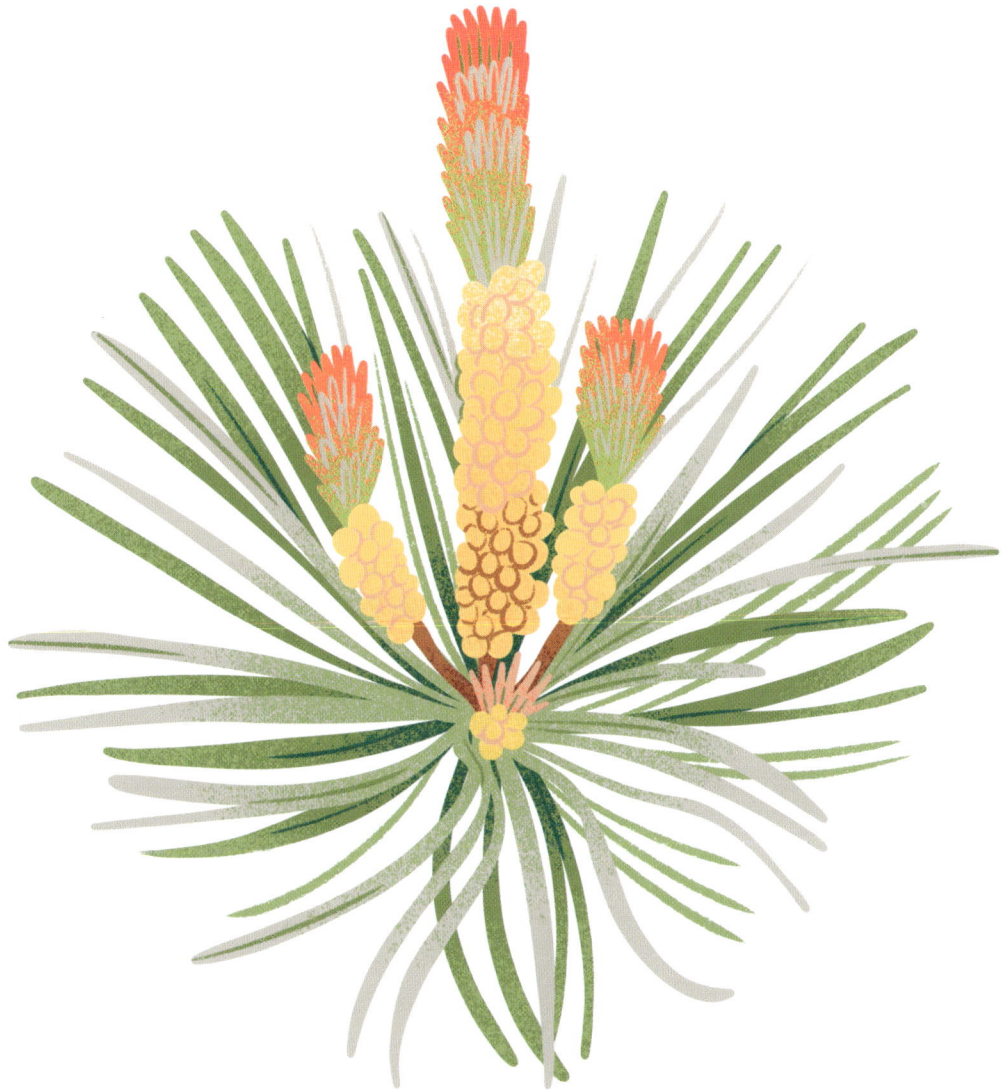

USDA hardiness zones: 3 to 8

Water: water young trees about 1 inch per week; mature trees need very little water

Light requirement: Full sun

Soil: grows best in soils in the 4.5 to 6.0 pH range, moist, and well-drained

Temperature: tolerates frost well

Wildlife notes: wild turkeys, quail, and squirrels readily eat the pine nuts

Pollinator friendly: wind-pollinated

Pests: bark beetles and borers

market, and classical music. And he often put these four things on repeat as conversation starters. So when a colleague told him about Vail and mentioned that it was a world-class destination—and despite the fact that I'd never known him to ski—he was all about the idea of exploring its runs, food, and wine scene.

It was 1981, and the TV in our condo had cable, which included a channel called MTV. I was obsessed with watching the intensively styled videos the musicians made for their songs. I will never forget giggling at Rod Stewart singing "Da Ya Think I'm Sexy" and Loverboy's red leather pants. I honestly would have been happy to just hole up in the condo, wrap myself up in a cozy blanket, and eat cereal all day. But when my mom and dad came out of their bedroom in matching neon jumpsuits, my dreams were dashed. Instead, we kids all got dumped at ski school to desperately try and learn to hold our skis in the "pizza" and "French fry" positions. All I could think about were my parents. I envisioned them swooshing down the slopes, pretending they didn't have kids, and sipping adult drinks by the cozy lodge fire. In the meantime, I was awkwardly learning to walk in ski boots.

At least I was warm. Growing up in Nebraska, you are taught from a very early age that if you dress appropriately you'll never be cold in the snow. Like my grandparents and parents before me, I walked "five miles in the snow each way" to school. The Nebraska blizzard of 1888 is memorialized in our state capitol, for Pete's sake—there's a mosaic of a woman holding a guide rope to help children safely walk home from school in the thick of it. As students, we all visited the state capitol every year for a field trip, so this story is truly emblazoned into our souls.

So as I was gliding up the ski lift in 1981, I was quite comfortable. I liked the chance to

relax, catch my breath. And it was up there I noticed the pine trees. I was flying over the tops of them. I tried to touch one with my ski and watched a bit of snow fall from its branches. I wished I could scoop up some snow in my mitten as I went by and eat it as I moved higher up the mountain. I kept looking at where the pine entered the snowpack and could not comprehend how far down below the surface the trunk might go. But at that moment, my eight-year-old self was higher than all the trees. I felt like a giant gracefully gliding above the whole world.

————————

My house today sits up on a little rise, and we have a few old pine trees here and there on the property. Each year, in the spring, I watch as the cutest little sprouts appear and cover the branches. They are bright green and remind me of spiky tufts of hair growing up toward the sky. Around the same time, the male pine cones form; they're plentiful and not woody like the female cones that appear in summer. They dangle down from the branches in groups, and if there is any sort of breeze, they shake off infinite amounts of pine pollen. The first year we lived here, I parked my car outside during this phenomenon (instead of in the garage) during a one-hour stop and drop between appointments. When I returned to my car, my mind couldn't quite comprehend what had happened. What was the thick yellow dust completely covering it?

Some researchers say pine pollen was used as early as the second century BC to treat various conditions. Today, pine pollen has been proven to be an effective treatment for hyperplasia of the prostate gland. Hyperplasia often starts with inflammation, or when a gene gets switched on and off. The result is an increase in cellular production, which leads to swelling or enlargement. This occurs in approximately 70 percent of men over the age of 60 and leads to the uncomfortable symptoms of bladder and sexual dysfunction.

Both men and women's testosterone levels can decrease with age, and pine pollen can be used to treat this as well. It is estimated that 10 grams of pine pollen contains 0.8 micrograms of testosterone, which can give our systems a boost if taken regularly. Perhaps it is the pine pollen's effect on the liver that supports more efficient hormone production and binding. In Chinese medicine, it is used to support the liver's detoxification pathway, cleansing the blood, and supporting overall function. One study proved that using pine pollen increased alcohol processing, which led to a quicker recovery time. Therefore, it has been proposed that pine pollen is a supportive medicinal for liver disease.

Improving athletic performance, supporting the immune system, and reducing daily fatigue are other reasons to consider taking pine pollen. Anytime you have an herbal with a high vitamin/mineral base you are going to receive a tonifying effect. Pine pollen is a good source of antioxidants including vitamin E, beta-carotene, selenium, and flavonoids. High antioxidants mean fewer free radicals in the body, which means less cellular damage overall. Vitamins and minerals are all utilized countless times in the millions of transactions that occur in the body on any given day. For example, a little bit of extra selenium supports the reproductive system, the thyroid, and fights infection. Having an adequate supply of every ingredient needed to successfully run our physical body's operating system is the difference between merely surviving and living with vitality.

Collecting pine pollen is a bit of a labor of love but a fun activity for a weekend afternoon. You'll know the male pine cones are ready for harvest when you give them a little tap and poofs of pollen puff out of them like little clouds of smoke. When you see that, you can simply twist off the pine cones one at a time, or snip the entire grouping off. While pine trees make an abundance of male cones, be cognizant not to overharvest from any one tree. Drop the cones in a big paper bag. Once you've collected the amount you need, take the harvest home to separate the pollen from the cone. The easiest way I've found to do this is to put 1 or 2 cups of cones into a mason jar and give a good shake for 3 to 5 minutes. The pollen will separate from the cone and then you can sift out any remaining bits of cone scales that will have peeled off during the agitation. Pine pollen is a very fine powder, so be sure to use a fine-mesh strainer when sifting. Store the pollen in a cool and dark place in an airtight container.

Pine Recipes

INDICATIONS

- Athletic performance
- Balance blood sugar
- Cholesterol
- Detoxifying enhancer
- Enlarged prostate
- Liver tonic
- Low testosterone
- Mental clarity
- Mood enhancer
- Skin health

Generally regarded as safe for all populations. Avoid if you have an allergy to any pine products.

PINE FLOWER ESSENCE

Flower essences treat our emotional side—a part of ourselves that we rarely take time to fully support. They are powerful medicines, indicated for when we seem to face the same obstacles in our lives over and over that result in suffering or the inability to move forward. I've used them for so many different things, from coping with the extreme shock of a car accident to relieving a child's recurring nightmares. Pine flower essence is also for when we make mistakes. Being human can be messy, and it is a constant learning experience. But when we persistently blame ourselves for our mistakes, as opposed to trying to understand and process them, we can be perpetually stuck in a cycle of shame. Pine helps to overcome that. It promotes self-compassion and reinforces that we are only human. As Morgan Richard Olivier once said; "You did the best you could with what you knew at the time. Don't let new wisdom lead you to condemn yourself over old struggles. Forgive yourself and move forward."

Items needed:
Large crystal bowl. (Glass can also work, but crystal is preferred; look at local garage sales for a vintage punch bowl someone is passing along—the perfect vessel.)
Storage bottle

Ingredients:
Fresh pine tips and needles
Spring water
High-quality brandy for preservation, if you plan to make a large batch and keep it for months/years

Choose a bright and clear sunny day to collect pine tips. Harvest them in the morning and put them into the crystal bowl.

Pour the spring water over the pine tips to completely cover with 2 to 3 inches of water. Using your hands, gently submerge the pine tips and needles.

Allow the pine to brew in full sun for 6 to 8 hours. It is believed that this process transfers the cellular energetic pattern of the plant into the water. After that time, gently strain out the pine tips and needles and pour the essence into a storage bottle.

Add brandy to preserve. I typically add a volume equal to ⅛ of my bottle size for preservation. So if you have an 8-oz. bottle, for example, add 1 oz. of brandy.

Take 10 drops whenever you feel it is needed.

PINE NEEDLE EGGNOG

Yup, that's right. Pine. Needle. Eggnog. Devon Young, better known by her Instagram handle @nittygrittymama, is an amazing author and herbalist. She, like me, loves the traditions of holidays and all of the blessed scents that go with them. Pass me a pine, cedar, or fir candle and I'm instantly transported to the winter holiday season. When I first read this recipe on her blog, I thought it said "consume for 2 hours." *Heck yeah!* was my first thought. But it actually says consume within 2 hours.

Items needed:
Saucepan
Mixing bowl
Whisk
Fine-mesh strainer
Stirring spoon
Hand mixer

Ingredients:
4 cups whole milk
4 eggs, yolks and whites separated
⅓ cup pine needles, cleaned and chopped
⅓ cup organic sugar
½ tsp. cinnamon
¼ tsp. fresh grated nutmeg
Optional: rum or bourbon, to taste

In a small saucepan over medium-low heat, bring the milk and pine needles to a low simmer. Do not boil. Simmer over low heat for 20 to 30 minutes.

Meanwhile, combine the egg yolks, sugar, and the spices. Whisk until light yellow and thick.

Pour milk/needle infusion through a fine-mesh strainer; discard needles. Slowly whisk the hot milk infusion into the yolk/sugar mixture.

Return the mixture to a small saucepan, pouring it through the fine-mesh strainer again. Over low heat, return the pot to a simmer and cook until the mixture thickens slightly and begins to coat the back of a spoon, about 5 minutes. Remove from the heat and chill completely.

Before serving, whip the egg whites to stiff peaks. Gently fold the whites into the eggnog. Add alcohol at this time if desired, according to your personal tastes. Ladle into a glass and serve. Consume within 2 hours.

Poplar

Populus candicans

Family: Salicaceae
Parts used: buds, bark
Medicinal actions:
bark: alterative, antiscorbutic, cathartic, discutient, diuretic, expectorant, stimulant, stomachic, tonic;
buds: diuretic, cathartic, demulcent, expectorant, nephritic, nutritive, stimulant, tonic
Native geography:
The Populus genus is now widely distributed globally and includes cottonwoods, aspens, and balsam poplars, but it is believed to have originated in the Northern Hemisphere.

Along the Sandy River delta, just east of Portland, Oregon, you'll find 1,500 acres of untouched land stretching from Portland to the Columbia River Gorge. It is one of those special places that offers nature at its purest self: peaceful, rugged, natural. I first discovered this environmental mecca when my friend asked if I wanted to go for a walk one Saturday. Being relatively new to Portland, I rarely turned down an invitation to do anything.

At the time, there was no designated parking lot. That would come years later as the site grew in popularity. We parked on a gravelly shoulder off the exit ramp from the highway, carefully opening the car door just enough to squeeze out. The tricky part was getting my friend's dog out safely because he knew where we were and was ready to spontaneously combust with excitement—about fifteen minutes into the drive, he had started to whine and pace in the back seat. Apparently he thought of this area as dog paradise.

After creeping along the side of the road, we finally ducked onto a trail, the dog was released from the leash, and we all relaxed. It was like no place I'd been before. The biodiversity was clearly evident from the multitude of different trees, plants, birds, and little critters like squirrels, chipmunks, and beavers. My friend shared that it had once been a flood plain with meadows, wetland, and bottomland forests, but like many natural spaces it had been impacted from short-term thinking such as deforestation and cattle grazing. Thankfully, the US Forest Service stepped in to acquire it in the early 1990s and has been supporting its rehabilitation ever since.

As we walked through a meadow of tall grass, I watched the dog leap and bounce like a deer through the woods. I could only see him each time he reached the apex of his jump, then he'd disappear again, hidden by the grasses. We continued down the trail as it entered a forest. The bright sunlight was suddenly gone and dark tree trunks took over the landscape. There was a wildness to this section of the preserve, something that made my heart beat a little faster. I noticed just a bit of sunlight here and there, but for the most part the scraggly branches that spread out from the trees created a dense canopy. It was as if they wanted to create their own secret world and suddenly I'd stepped into it.

As I approached a group of a few similar trees clumped together, I immediately noticed their budding tips. Poplar buds emerge tightly wound and encased in resin, which gives them a look like they've been lacquered several times over. Their color is unique—a purplish mocha brown that lightens just a bit as the buds prepare to leaf out. That day, I pinched a bud and rubbed it between my thumb and forefinger knowing I'd elicit one of my favorite smells on earth. A light floral fragrance that has an undertone of honey and musk. My friend came up, along with the dog, both curious what I was up to. I pointed out the medicine growing all around us and explained how to use it. We hatched a plan to return the following week to wildcraft.

We continued walking along, talking and taking moments of silence to soak all the beauty in until we found ourselves on the banks of the river. The dog came sprinting

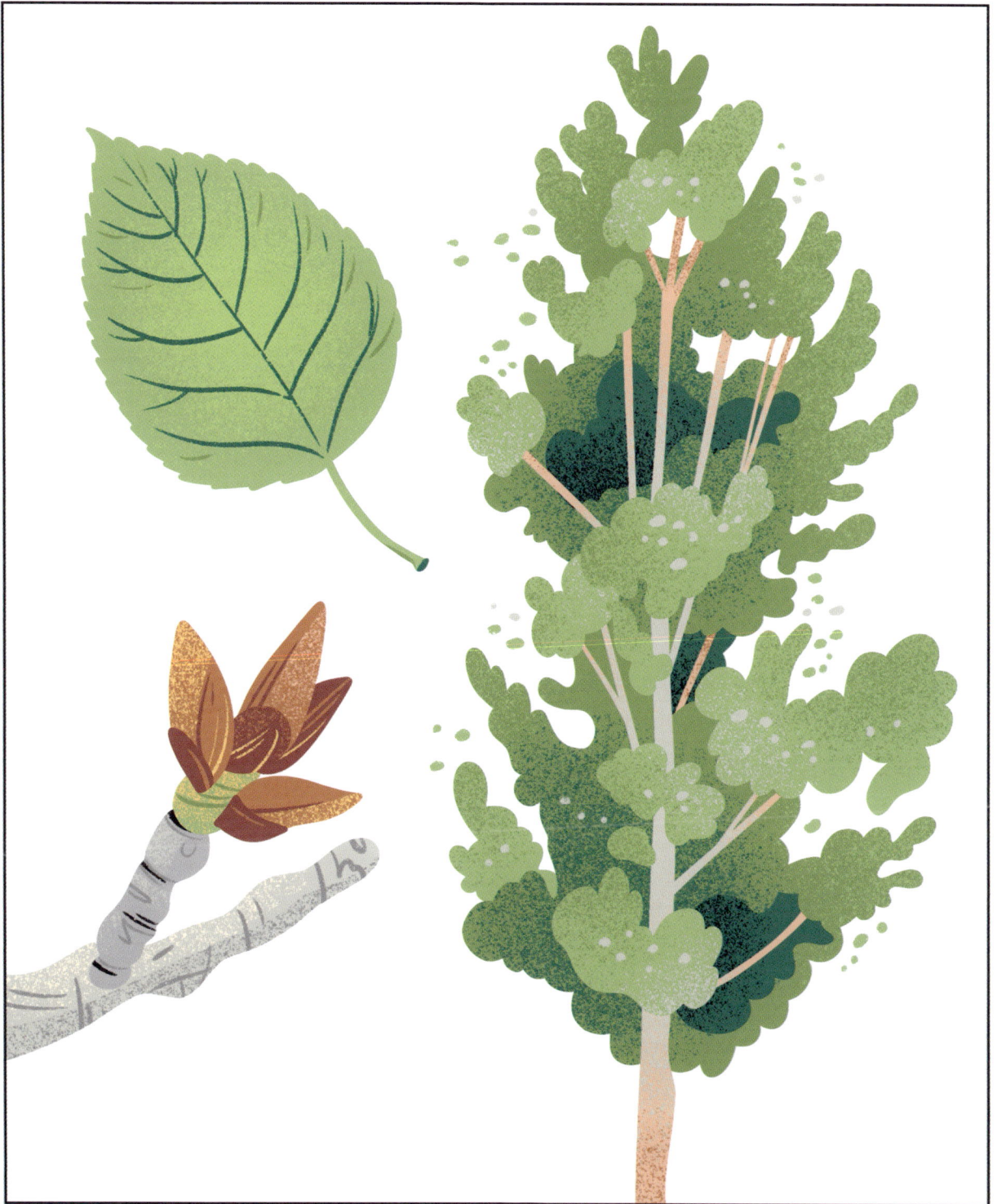

PLANT DATA
USDA hardiness
zones: 4 to 9
Water: poplars need
moist soil to thrive, but
will show self-imposed
reactions to drought
such as limiting leaf
growth and dropping
leaves early
Light requirement:
full sun
Soil: preference for
moist, well-drained,
humus-rich fertile soil
that is slightly acidic
Temperature: hardy to
-20°F
Wildlife notes: deer,
elk, and bird populations
have tended to increase
when poplars are planted
Pollinator friendly:
wind-pollinated, but
bees love the resin
Pests: canker and
wetwood, leaf-feeding
caterpillars, leaf beetles,
cottony-cushion scales,
and mealybugs

past us from behind and jumped in the water with a huge leap. As I looked to the right and then the left, I noticed poplar trees lining the Columbia River. Their long, straight trunks stood sentry on the bank of the river like a row of warriors defending their home. It made me think of the Chehalis—a tribe in Washington that considers poplar to have a spirit all its own. In part this is probably because the trees are known to shake their leaves even when there is no wind. When we finally forced ourselves to walk back to the car, I turned and noticed that all of the leaves were shaking as if waving us goodbye.

———————

My personal calendar is marked by seasons, with indications of when and where I need to harvest certain medicinals. I often think about planting a medicinal garden on a grand scale, but there are some wild harvesting trips I would miss too much. One of those is in search of poplar buds in late winter—just when the January days are sunny but you still need to dress with a coat and scarf in the morning.

Tightly woven buds appear on the tips of branches. They are a deep mahogany color and as temperatures rise, you can see suspended resin droplets on their exterior. Here in Oregon we have copious groves of poplar trees. This, in combination with our ever-increasing winter winds, makes it easy to find downed trees and branches that are still producing buds. It always amazes me how a tree can fall over in the winter yet still produce spring leaves and flowers.

Once you find a tree or branch with buds, pluck them right off and put them into a paper bag or basket. The timing of this is particular: you want the buds to be fully developed, right on the brink of loosening up.

Once they begin to open, harvesting becomes a sticky job, and I think you lose some of the medicinal properties to oxidation. I typically let the buds dry inside for 24 hours before processing them into oil. Poplar takes a bit longer to cook than typical herbal oils. I also have a designated slow cooker just for poplar because the resin makes it virtually impossible to clean. Cook it on warm for 72 hours with a lid just a smidge ajar.

Once you learn the medicinal qualities of a tree, it can be difficult not to think about them every time you encounter a given species in the woods. Such is the case with poplar/cottonwood trees for me, anyway. As winter winds down, I find myself almost subconsciously watching for the tightly wound poplar buds to emerge as I take walks. As the layers upon layers of potential new life come into view, you can trust that winter is ending and the promise of spring is coming. And the fragrance is like no other; perhaps the scent alerts me to the buds' arrival. When you pluck a bud that's the color of sangria and give it a gentle squeeze between your fingers, a deep red, resinous oil escapes and rolls down your hand. This is the oil of poplar, a coveted medicine of herbalists because it has been used for a plethora of ailments. Foraging poplar at the right times of year will keep your medicine cabinet stocked with remedies for everyday afflictions, much like our ancestors did.

Much of poplars' use is centered around muscle aches and pains, and it is definitely very good at treating those. I tend to rub it on everything as a panacea of sorts, probably mostly out of habit. But when I strain my back or my knee acts up, reaching for the poplar oil usually does the trick. Poplar contains salicin, a natural pain-reducing agent similar to aspirin. This acts as an anti-inflammatory and can help with body aches, joint pains, fever, and headache. When poplar is ingested, the salicin is converted into salicylic acid—this also contributes to moderating inflammation by downregulating prostaglandins.

Poplar's inner bark also has medicinal value. I harvest this from downed branches or snip small twigs off a tree to avoid damaging a healthy tree. I recommend the bark for respiratory complaints, particularly when there is excessive inflammation of the lungs with a little thicker phlegm present. This includes bronchitis, pleurisy, and pneumonia but also the common cough and cold. Because there is a counterirritant quality to poplar, it also increases circulation as it has an affinity to the respiratory system. This can be helpful to usher in new blood and lymph cells when trying to fight infection. In conjunction with internal use, you can apply the topical oil to the chest for additional support.

Poplar is also an antiseptic and a natural immune booster. Honeybees are drawn to the tree for this specific reason, and it therefore becomes a component of propolis. Propolis is a bee-manufactured resin made from plant exudates, beeswax, and their saliva. When a colony is under the threat of infection, they will make more as a way to boost their collective immune system. It is one example of bees using medicinals just like us.

Poplar Recipes

_____

INDICATIONS

- Arthritis
- Backache
- Bronchitis
- Colds
- Cough
- Headache
- Pleurisy
- Pneumonia
- Prostaglandin, decrease
- Rheumatism
- Wound healing

Generally regarded as safe for all populations. Do not use if you have an aspirin allergy. Avoid if honey allergy is present.

POPLAR BUD PAIN RELIEF SALVE

Poplar bud harvest is one of my favorite times of year. It not only signals the coming end of winter, but the harvest is typically done after a day or two of warm winter weather. Walking in the warm sunshine after weeks of relentless rain feels like a rebirth, or the emergence from a cocoon. Recipe makes 10 1-oz. tins.

Items needed:
Dedicated salve saucepan
Metal spoon
Wax paper
Toothpicks
10 1-oz. tins for storage

Ingredients:
10 oz. poplar oil
3.5 oz. melted beeswax
50 to 60 drops of ginger essential oil

Please refer to the description in this chapter for how to wild-harvest the poplar buds and make the oil needed for this recipe. Once you've strained the poplar buds from the oil, transfer the oil to a saucepan and add the beeswax.

Line up your tins on top of wax paper; this is mainly in case you spill. Add 5 to 6 drops of ginger essential oil to each tin.

Keeping the heat on low and stirring regularly, completely melt the beeswax. The suggested ratio of oil to beeswax in this recipe will keep the salve soft and spreadable. If you want something a little more firm, which is helpful when traveling to hotter climates, add a bit more beeswax.

Carefully pour the liquid into the tins and give each a quick stir with a toothpick to combine the liquid with the essential oil.

Allow to cool fully without the lid before sealing.

POPLAR LUNG-EASE TINCTURE

This recipe is a surefire treatment for those who are battling with either a chronic or sudden-onset respiratory infection. When taken dutifully, it often clears up the condition within just a few days.

Items needed:
8-oz. glass mason jar
Wax paper
Strainer
Storage bottle
Two 4-oz. dropper bottles

Ingredients:
Poplar bark, freshly wildcrafted
Organic cane alcohol
1 oz. apple cider vinegar
1 oz. vegetable glycerin

Make a trip to the woods, or your backyard if you've got your own poplar tree, and harvest some fresh inner bark, enough to fill the 8-oz. jar.

Next, add the organic cane alcohol, filling the jar ¾ of the way. Add 1 oz. of apple cider vinegar and 1 oz. of vegetable glycerin.

Place the metal lid on top of the jar and place a large square piece of wax paper over that before putting on the screw band. Next, give it a good shake for 1 minute.

Label and place in a cool, dark place for 2 weeks, ensuring that you are shaking it every day.

Strain after the 2 weeks and transfer it into the 2 4-oz. dropper bottles.

I typically recommend 1 to 2 dropperfuls every 2 to 3 hours for 24 to 48 hours, then once 3 times per day for 2 weeks.

Quaking Aspen

Populus tremuloides

Family: Salicaceae
Parts used: bark, buds, resin
Medicinal actions: anti-inflammatory, antiscorbutic, balsamic, diaphoretic, diuretic, expectorant, febrifuge, purgative, stomachic, tonic, vermifuge
Native geography: North America

"Let's hit the road," said my friend. "We can see the fall foliage." That was all it took. "Hell yes!" I said. I recall having felt bogged down by adulting just when he asked, having moved into that phase of life subtly and imperceptibly. I needed to get out of Dodge, breathe some fresh air, and see the quaking aspens turn gold. At twenty-five, I had followed the generally prescribed course society encourages toward "success," and I had no idea that deviating was an option. As a middle--class Midwesterner, I'd been a good girl on the outside. I'd gotten good grades, applied to college, gotten in, and gotten a job to help pay the way. I ended up going to the University of Nebraska, but had also applied to Colorado College, TCU, and the University of California, Santa Barbara. I didn't really want to go to Nebraska. I'd daydreamed about a completely different life in those other places, but in the end cost and convenience won out.

After four years and exploring several majors, I ended up with a mishmash of a dual degree in biochemistry and English. I took twenty credits both terms my senior year because I just needed to be finished. Get out of college, get out of Nebraska. I felt it in my bones. My soul was undernourished. I basically ran straight to Colorado after graduation, snowboarding and just enjoying living in a mountainous ski town. At age twenty-three, I was officially on my own, a state away from my family, and beginning what I now call my "baby adulting phase." I was working two jobs but I was young, which basically equates to being able to burn both ends of the candle and still wake up feeling happy. If my shift ended at 10 p.m., I could easily hang out until 1 a.m. or 2 a.m. and easily get up for an 8 a.m. shift the next day. I could exist on ramen, cookies, and bread for weeks until payday. I was finally free from the mental constraints of what I was supposed to be doing and able to live the way I'd always dreamed about. I was poor but happy, able to make rent and not go hungry—all while living at 9,500 feet. It was magical, chaotic, and definitely difficult at times—all the things life should be in your early twenties. Toward the end of the ski season, a black-diamond mogul trail got the best of me, the jobs dried up, and I ended up back home in Nebraska.

A year passed; I was in a rut. I was the registrar at a business college, a school filled with people in my age range, all of us trying to figure out what this life thing was about. Previously, I'd been managing a café, but for some reason I thought I needed to "move up" in the adulting world and applied for the registrar job—I quickly realized it wasn't necessarily ideal for an adventurous, creative, twenty-five-year-old Aries. While working there, my friend Peter told me about Pando, a quaking aspen grove in Utah. It isn't considered a forest, despite looking like one, because every trunk of the 40,000 quaking aspen trees that we see above ground is connected by a single 80,000-year-old root system. It's a clone, one of the world's single largest organisms. I added seeing it to my bucket list.

A short time later, my friend tempted me to take a break and hit the road. The goal was clear: we were on the road to Pando. We had to

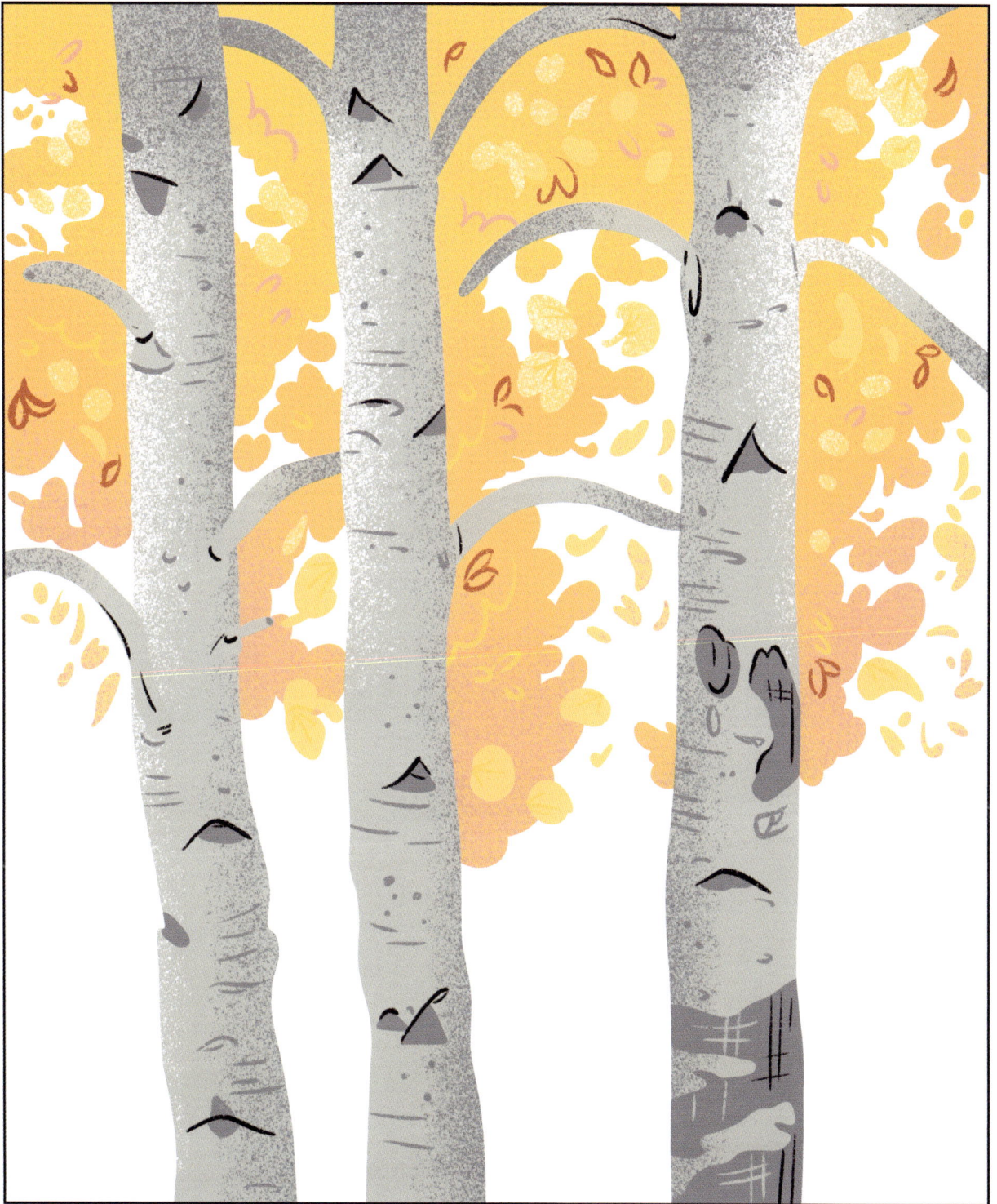

**USDA hardiness
zones:** 2 to 8
Water: water deeply
every 2 to 4 weeks
Light requirement:
full sun
Soil: well-drained, and
with a touch of acidity
Temperature: not tolerant of hot summers
Wildlife notes: wood-
pecker species like
flickers and sapsuckers
prefer to nest in aspen
when possible
Pollinator friendly:
wind-pollinated, but
bees and wasps are at-
tracted to spring flowers
Pests: aphids, blight ink-
spot disease, oystershell
scale

see this ancient tree family for ourselves and quickly agreed that the thirteen-hour drive would be well worth it. Plus, road-tripping was one of our love languages. We both craved them and had taken many together, frequently, for many years. As a master of making mixtapes, he was the DJ. He made a sequence of tapes to accompany us as we cruised down the road in his white Caprice classic. I was in charge of navigation.

As we drove through Nebraska, across Colorado, and into Utah, I watched the landscape change before my eyes. I also watched for "tree spirits," which is what I like to call images that look like people or animals within the trees—it's similar to seeing things in the clouds. I actually used to see them more clearly before I had LASIK. It was as if they revealed themselves only through the faultiness of my sight, but as I age and my eyes decline again, they are returning more and more. Perhaps it is my mind bending to my desire to want to see something, but I like to think of it as the tree spirits showing up to say hello. You may think I'm a silly old woman, but I choose to live in a world where magic is just right around the corner.

At about a mile past Fish Lake on Highway 25, we began to wonder if we'd found it. There is no sign where Pando starts, just a slow realization that you've arrived when you hit mile marker 6 and you begin to see the trees. We slowed down and pulled the car into a turnout so we could get out and walk through this natural wonder. It was a bright, blue-sky day and the sun was hitting the brilliant yellow leaves in a way that made them look like they were illuminated from the inside. I can only describe it by saying that it looked like Pando's aura was burning bright. It felt magical to be touching and witnessing something so deeply old and connected to the earth. We walked among the trees for hours,

running our fingers along the tree trunks and collecting leaves like you might collect seashells at the beach. We had to drag ourselves back to the car when the light began to fade, feeling sad that we had to leave our new friend. As the wind picked up the leaves began to quake, a sure signal that our friend was waving goodbye.

———————

Similar to the balsam poplar, the quaking aspen has resinous buds and medicinal bark. But they are often used in different ways. Most herbalists consider balsam poplar buds to be superior in regards to anti-inflammatory effects for sore muscles and joints, whereas quaking aspen buds have traditionally been infused to make a tea to treat the upper respiratory system. We drink it to soothe coughs and clear the sinuses, and it makes a good gargle for a sore throat. It's also a highly effective treatment for fever, which may indicate that it mobilizes the circulatory system.

Historically, herbalists set a precedent for understanding how and when to use quaking aspen. The notion is to use it when there is a hyperstimulation event occurring in the body—when the sympathetic nervous system is always on, not allowing our body to enter the "rest and digest" phase, or the parasympathetic to be in balance. When one or the other of these two systems is dominating our daily lives, things can go south quite quickly. One example is our digestive system: ideally, our parasympathetic nervous system turns on before we eat. Once turned on, it sends messages to our mouth (mouth waters) and to our stomach to prepare for the arrival of food (hydrochloric acid production begins). If our sympathetic state is constantly under stress, these preparation steps never occur. You can eat without HCL and digestion enzymes armed and ready, but you will not break down your food as effectively or efficiently. This often leads to inflammation and lower nutrient absorption of the food you eat.

Quaking aspen is marked for having an effect on the sympathetic state and can be considered for many different "hyper" conditions. It's often recommended for an overactive bladder or kidneys under stress. If there is no general urge to urinate but you find that the moment you need to complete a task or speak to someone a sudden and violent urge arises, that is what we call bladder nervousness. In that moment the overactive sympathetic state kicks in a reflex, stimulating the brain to have a bladder response. Another example is if the digestive system is never relaxed. As a result, the colon will have excess peristalsis, or contraction waves, leading to chronic diarrhea. This in turn results in the loss of nutrient uptake, causing a loss in vitality.

Utilizing quaking aspen to calm or reset the sympathetic nervous system can recalibrate physical systems and bring them back into balance. Now, if you are one of the people who drinks lattes throughout the day to keep your full-throttle switch on, this will be an uphill battle. But if you've shifted your diet and feel as if you are still in constant overdrive, this might be a good medicine to consider.

Historically, quaking aspen was considered a famine food—a plant that people ate only in times of severe food shortage. Knowing which plants are nutrient powerhouses is always a good thing to have in your back pocket. The inner bark and catkins (the cylindrical flower that hangs down) can be eaten fresh or cooked. For a carbohydrate source, you can cut long strips of the inner bark, dry it, grind it into flour, and make bread. The springtime buds, before they are opened, can also be consumed and are good sources of vitamin A, calcium, and fiber.

Quaking aspens are a wonderful addition to a home yard, especially if you love to watch their heart-shaped leaves shake in the bright sun of fall. They have alternate leaves that are ovate and finely toothed, and they grow on tiny petioles that allow them to move so freely in the wind. This is what makes them look like they are trembling, or "quaking."

Quaking Aspen Recipes

INDICATIONS

- Bedsores
- Bladder weakness
- Chills and fever
- Colds
- Coughs
- Cystitis
- Diarrhea
- Digestive tonic
- Hyperthyroid
- Kidney tonic
- Nervousness
- Sore throats
- Sinus
- Tremors
- Wounds

Generally regarded as safe for all populations. Contraindicated for use with aspirin.

PAIN TWIG

Quaking aspen is truly a forest woman's dream. This tree's bounty seems endless. When you are out in the wild and in need, quaking aspen has a lot to offer.

Items needed:
Pruning shears

Ingredients:
One quaking aspen twig

If you're feeling a headache come on, or have a toothache or other type of discomfort, clip a small twig from a quaking aspen tree and chew on it like you might chew on a toothpick.

NATURAL SUNSCREEN

If you find yourself out in the woods on a sunny day and realize you forgot to put on sunscreen, look for a quaking aspen. The leaves and trunk should be coated in a fine powder. This powder is created as the bark sheds its old cells. As and after it does this, the powdery residue is left behind. This powder has traditionally been used as an effective sunscreen. Simply wipe some from the tree and apply it to your face.

Or, if you've got dry, cracked hands in the winter, rub some of the tree's powdery substance on them. It helps to seal up cracks and splits. It's good for tiny cuts, too, as well as the pain and swelling of insect bites and stings.

TENSION TAMER HEADACHE RELIEF TEA

Unfortunately, I'm no stranger to migraines. For me they come from various sources, such as hormones and food sensitivities, but they can also be triggered by stress. When I'm feeling noticeably tense, I reach for this tea.

Items needed:
Saucepan

Ingredients:
1 tbsp. quaking aspen bark
1 tbsp. white willow bark
1 tsp. lavender flowers
2 tsp. mint
4 cups water

Bring the water to boil in the saucepan. Add the quaking aspen and white willow bark and simmer for 5 minutes, uncovered. Turn off the heat. Add the mint, cover, and let steep for 10 minutes. Finally, add the lavender, cover, and let steep for 3 minutes.

Strain and enjoy.

Sitka Spruce

Picea sitchensis,
Picea abies

Family: Pinaceae
Parts used: young
shoots, needles
Medicinal actions:
analgesic, anti-
inflammatory, antimi-
crobial, antiseptic, antispasmodic, astringent,
calmative, diaphoretic,
expectorant, immune
tonic
Native geography:
the Pacific Northwest;
they grow from Alaska
to Northern California
and prefer to stay close
to the ocean and its
salty shores

When I first moved to my property, I noticed a small tree way down in the corner of the lot, by the road. I remember thinking, "What a funny place to plant a tree." It was all alone at the bottom of my field. I grabbed my tree identification book—dogeared and packed with leaf, twig and flower samples I've collected over the years—and marched down to get a better look. I was pleasantly surprised to identify it as a Sitka spruce, a prized medicinal. It didn't appear very old, but it looked well established, which meant it would soon start to grow fast.

Through the years, I've been told bits and pieces about where my Sitka tree came from. The version I like best, and therefore have adopted, is about a man who lived in this area years before. As a tribute, and before all the fences that now separate us were built, he'd gone up and down this stretch of agricultural zone and planted thirty of these trees in hopes they'd stand tall, forever, among all the Christmas tree farms that inhabit this land. Supposedly this tribute originated after a visit to the Olympic National Park in Washington, where he'd come across, by pure chance, the oldest Sitka spruce tree in the United States.

When I hear someone make judgments like "the oldest tree," I pause. In our busy day-to-day lives, it can be easy to disregard a statement without considering its implications. Luckily, I like to ponder these types of things. I immediately started to research Sitka spruces. They have true resilience, are known to stand the test of time, and the one in Washington is estimated to be between 800 and 1,000 years old. To think about what human events this tree has witnessed through the centuries is a fun pastime for me. It grows close to Lake Quinault, perhaps nourished from the streams emerging from that body of water. How many fires and floods has this tree endured? How many birds have nested in its branches? How many genera-tions of the Cayuse, Umatilla, and Walla Walla peoples had touched this tree over the years? I wanted to sit underneath it and feel its ancient wisdom. Maybe if I got close enough, I thought, it would whisper secrets of the past in my ear.

I was so intrigued that just a few weeks later I packed up the kids and drove north to see it for myself. I'd learned that this Washington Sitka was considered a "pioneer" tree of the Pacific Northwest because it was one of the first to arrive in this area after the glacier recession following the last ice age. As we drove north, my thoughts drifted to wondering if someone had planted this partic-ular tree. And if so, who? Or maybe a bird had dropped a seed and it self-germinated. Sitkas appear along the West Coast, from Northern California up to Alaska. Even the wind could have carried the seed for miles and miles to this pristine destination.

Years before, my kids and I had visited Oregon's biggest Sitka, but it wasn't as old as the one in Washington. I have a photo of us with our arms stretched around the trunk, trying our best to touch each other's fingers. It was struck by lightning in 1967 and had survived, but in 2007 a winter storm with high winds

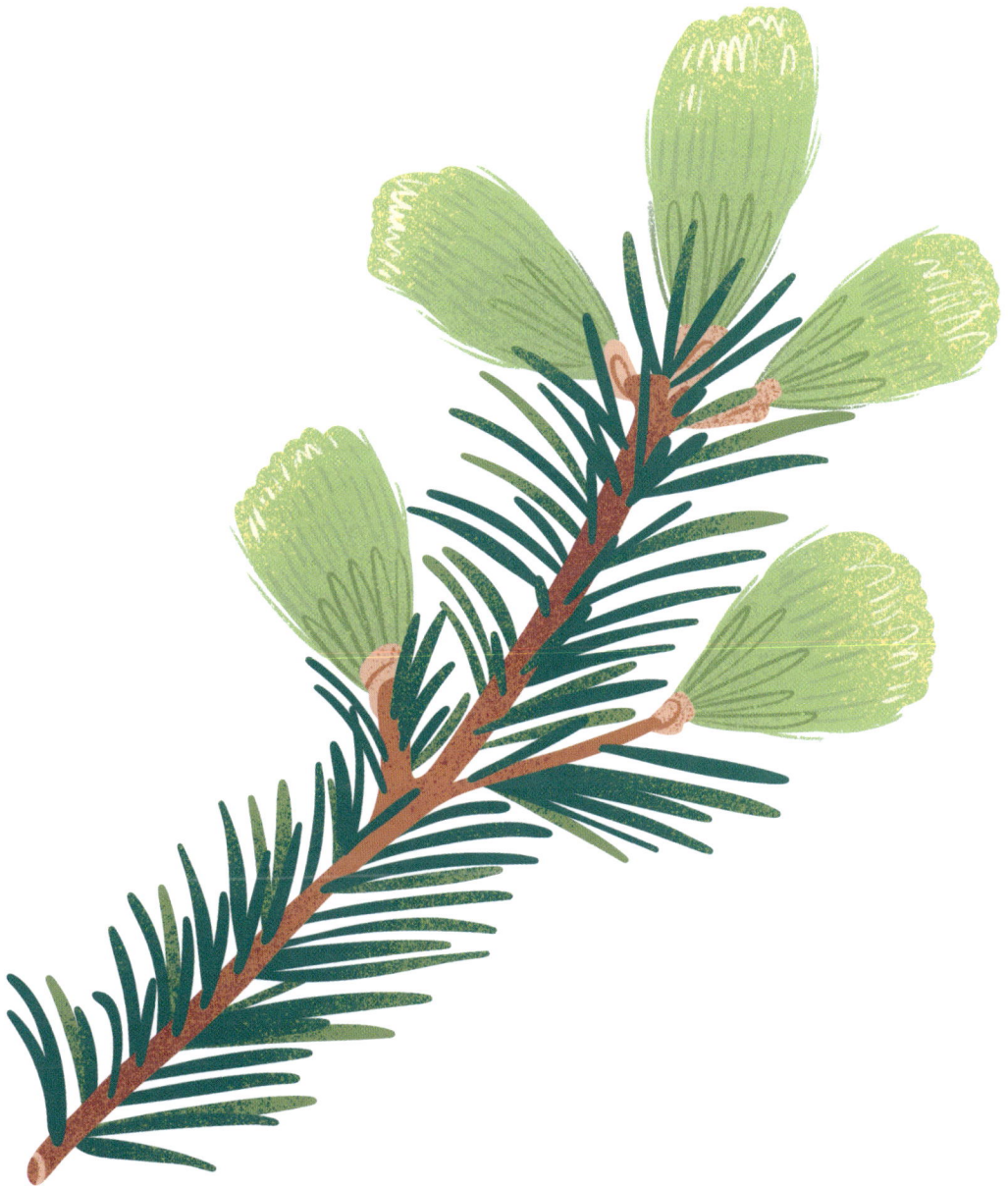

PLANT DATA

USDA hardiness zones: 6 to 8

Water: Sitkas need a lot of water and humidity to be happy; a minimum of 5 inches of water in the summer

Light requirement: full sun

Soil: strong affinity for soils high in calcium, magnesium, and phosphorus

Temperature: prefers cold and wind to summer droughts

Wildlife notes: dense foliage provides cover from the wind and rain for larger mammals; birds of prey like perching up high, and smaller birds such as crossbill, tree creeper, coal tit, and siskin use it for nesting

Pollinator friendly: wind-pollinated

Pests: broom rust, green spruce aphid, needle cast, various beetle, white pine weevil

snapped the tree. It felt like losing a grandparent, and many of us went to pay our respects and mourn the loss of an incredible elder.

As we passed Lake Quinault, I noticed I was chewing gum vigorously while looking at my map and the mile markers to ensure I was going the right way. I grew antsy with excitement, which spilled over to my kids, who in turn also became excited, feeding off my energy. I kept changing the radio station, and when a song came on we all liked we'd sing at the top of our lungs as an attempt to release what was building up. My kids were bouncing up and down by the time I finally saw the sign for the Sitka and turned off into a parking lot. Almost before I could park the car, my kids burst out and ran toward the tree as if it were a dear old friend. It stood 191 feet tall, and its trunk was nearly 50 inches in diameter. We all froze to take it all in. "Approximately 1,000 years old," the informative plaque read. Again, I was dumbfounded at the idea of touching a living thing that had lived so long. How far down did the roots go? I thought they might reach most of the way to the center of the earth.

As we all slowly walked around the base of the tree, we had to climb up and down, often with uneven footing, because of its "flare" base. It was as if we were climbing on a dinosaur's back, with all its reptilian ridges and ravines. Up higher, on the straight trunk, the dark-purple bark was scaly and rough. I slid my hand around to brace myself and a bit of pitch stuck to my thumb. I pulled out a small jar and collected a few teaspoons of the sticky goo to use in my next wound salve. I tucked this precious gift into my pocket, and we each found a place to settle in among the base's deep grooves. My daughter contemplated whether she could climb it while my son began to draw the tree in his notebook. I wanted to tell the tree all about its distant

relative living on my farm. I wondered, if by some pure genetic magic, how tightly woven their DNA might be. As I leaned back onto its curved trunk, I pondered this and a thousand other things about coincidences, landscapes, and history. "A thousand years old," I whispered aloud. Then, I closed my eyes and waited to receive the stories it was ready to share with me.

———————

Sitkas can be identified from other conifers of the region because they typically have a flared base, making it look as if the trunk is penetrating down into the ground rather than rising up out of its roots. While a Sitka technically has leaves, in conifers they are usually referred to as needles or scales. The Sitka's needles are stiff and sharp. From far away they look deep green, but as you approach you can see they have a blue hue. Each needle is four-sided and they are attached spirally, making them look like a bottle brush. They usually lay flat in a cross section that points both perpendicular to the branch twig and toward the tip. New spring sprigs are 1 to 2 inches long—and beautiful when spread out on a tray or soaking in a mason jar.

Sitkas are a great tree to have around for all the things that bother us during the winter months. During the summer and for part of the fall, we still have our windows open, allowing for fresh air to sweep in and circulate. Once temperatures drop, windows get closed and for some do not open again until spring. Once our inside home environment is closed off, it is easier for bacteria and viruses to settle in and spread. Sitka needles make a slightly sweet tea that is helpful in reducing coughs, colds, and the flu. It promotes a gentle sweating of the skin as well, to help flush out the illness without leaving the patient exhausted. You can also add it to a bath when you aren't feeling well and the heat will release its aromatic oils into the steam. This creates a medicinal inhalation treatment as you are soaking, going right to the source of common colds: the respiratory tract. Or add Sitka needles to a pot of hot water for facial/nasal steam upon rising and/or before bed to help clear out congestion and mucous. Chew a bit of a fresh shoot to cleanse out the mouth and soothe the throat. You can also use Sitka needles to make a gargle for laryngitis, strep throat, or swollen tonsils.

There is a relatively high vitamin C content in fresh Sitka sprouts and needles, but it has been determined that in order to get the highest vitamin concentration from them, freeze-drying is best. Freeze-dried needles contain roughly 30 percent more vitamins than standard drying or even the fresh material. They also contain a good supply of magnesium, potassium, vitamin A, and E.

Adding Sitka to the bath is also good to relieve back aches caused by colds and flus or from overwork. The Sitka relaxes muscle tension and can help to reduce pain. An aromatic bath is a great way to end a long day of working in the garden or on the farm. I suggest putting the shoots and needles into a muslin bag before adding it to the bath, but I'll be the first to admit, I find pleasure in seeing them floating freely as well.

The gum and resin of Sitka are a great resource if needed for wound healing and to keep a wound clean in order to prevent infection. While I have no firsthand experience with it, thankfully, it is said that the gum from the fresh shoots, when placed into the eyes, is to be used if suffering from snow blindness.

Sitka Spruce Recipes

INDICATIONS

- Backache
- Bronchitis
- Colds
- Cough
- Fever
- Flu
- Snow blindness
- Toothache
- Wounds

*Generally regarded as
 safe for all populations.*

SITKA-TIP SYRUP

An easy recipe to have on hand and ready for the winter to fight sore throats and laryngitis.

Simply make alternating layers of fresh Sitka tips and brown sugar in a quart-size mason jar, in approximately equal parts. I tend to start with sugar, then tips, then sugar and so on until I reach the top ¼ of the jar.

Close the jar with a lid and let the mixture sit for 8 weeks, preferably in a warm spot.

Then, gently warm the liquid in a saucepan. Strain.

Store this syrup in a clean bottle in the fridge for up to 4 months

CITRUS SITKA ICING

A light and bright addition to cookies and cakes for any time of year.

Items needed:
Spice grinder or herb grinder
Citrus juicer
Small mixing bowl
Stirring spoon

Ingredients:
3 tbsp. ground sitka spruce needles
1 to 1½ cup icing sugar
1 tbsp. freshly squeezed orange juice
Splash of heavy cream

To get finely ground needles, you'll need an automated nut/herb/seed grinder or spice grinder. This takes a little bit of patience at first, as it seems to grow and get fluffy, but stay the course and it will grind down.

Using a citrus juicer, squeeze half of an orange into a bowl.

Put the ground needles into the bowl and begin adding icing sugar, one tablespoon at a time, until you get a fine-looking paste.

Next, add the orange juice and splash of heavy cream and mix well. If you need to add a bit more icing sugar at this point, that is okay. Mix until you reach the icing consistency you prefer, thicker or thinner.

You can put this on top of anything you'd like—a fresh batch of shortbread cookies, or as a nice glaze on top of a lemon loaf or even over pancakes.

SITKA EVERYDAY CRACKERS

Beware, these are very addicting. They are great with cheese, dips, salami, jam … pretty much anything that can fit on a cracker.

Items needed:
Mixing bowl
Whisk
Parchment paper
Rolling pin
Pastry wheel or knife
Cookie sheet

Ingredients:
1 cup white unbleached all-purpose flour
½ cup whole wheat flour, or tapioca or flax meal
1 tbsp. finely chopped Sitka spruce tips
1 tsp. granulated sugar
1 tsp. Himalayan sea salt
¼ tsp. black pepper
2 tbsp. olive oil
½ to ¾ cup water, plus more for brushing

Preheat the oven to 475° F.

Whisk together both flours, salt, sugar, and Sitka tips. Then stir in the oil and water and mix until fully combined. The dough shouldn't be wet, but it should be sticky.

Place a piece of parchment paper the same size as your cookie sheet down on your workspace. Sprinkle the parchment with flour.

Once you get your dough into a nice shape, begin to roll it out. Flour your rolling pin to stop the dough from sticking to the pin.

The thinner the dough, the crisper the cracker. You are aiming for about ⅛-inch thickness.

Once rolled out, trim the sides; the edges often get too thin and then they burn in the oven. For pretty crackers, use a pastry wheel to cut the dough into rectangles.

Next, brush a light coating of water on top, then sprinkle the crackers with salt.

Using a fork, poke a few holes into each cracker to help them bake evenly.

Transfer the entire parchment paper to your cookie sheet and bake for 12 to 20 minutes, depending on your oven. Keep an eye on them; when they look golden and delicious, they are probably done.

White Willow

*Salix alba, Salix fragilis,
Salix nigra*

Family: Salicaceae
Parts used: bark
Medicinal actions:
anodyne, anti-
inflammatory, antipyretic,
antiseptic, astringent,
diaphoretic, diuretic,
febrifuge, tonic
Native geography:
Europe, central Asia, and
northern Africa. Europe-
an settlers brought white
willow to the United
States in the 1700s and
now it grows in eastern
North America, from
New Brunswick and
southern Ontario, west
to Minnesota, and south
to northern Florida
and Texas.

As a kid, my best friend was a white willow. I grew up on South Seventeenth Street in Lincoln, Nebraska. We lived in a two-story, gray house in a neighborhood filled with old people. They probably weren't actually that old, but they seemed like it to us and there definitely weren't any kids to play with nearby. All of the kids lived over in Woodshire, a neighborhood built around Woodshire Park. It was two blocks from my house, but it was like another world. It was truly a park, not a playground. There weren't any swing sets or slides where groups of kids would gather to play tag or the floor is lava. It was a park in the sense of giant trees, beautiful green grassy slopes in the summer, and endless snow tunnels in the winter. It was where we all met for the Fourth of July to share prize-winning pies and every type of Midwestern salad known to woman. It was where we all had our graduation parties with little pop-up tents and balloons, our heels sinking into the aerated grass. It was where I had my first kiss—a peck on my cheek that was all innocence and the sweetness and from an earnest boy. It was where we all ended up on snow days. Back then Nebraska had epic snow days, sometimes feet upon feet of it falling overnight. Once we were bundled up and resembling Randy from the 1983 movie *A Christmas Story*, we would grab our sleds and waddle out into the tundra for hours on end with the promise of warm hot chocolate waiting for us when we returned.

Despite there being more kids in Woodshire to play with, there were still no girls. It was always me and Kevin, Brooks,

his younger brother Hugh, Mike, Chris, and Vikram. A great group, but I longed for something that seemed to be missing, and this is where willow began to fill the gap. Most of the kid activity took place right in the middle of the park, but my favorite spot was at the north end, where a giant weeping willow lived. Its long branches were always gently swaying from side to side like pen- dulums. It felt very feminine to me, this swaying, like gentle hips and a torso moving to music I couldn't hear. My generation had grown up with Shel Silverstein's *The Giving Tree*, and although that concerned an apple tree, the branches in the book so resembled my willow that it was nearly impossible not to personify this tree, too. I would rush toward the tendrils, slipping my hands between them and parting them, pretending there was another world waiting for me on the other side. Because the tendrils were so long, they created a screen from the outside world once inside. A screen of bright spring green that hid me and my secrets away from everyone else. By April of each year, thou- sands of fairy-size leaves appeared. When it rained, individual raindrops would sit perfectly on the center of each leaf. A woolly screen of deeper green showed up through- out the summer and fall. The only time I had company inside its branches was when we would play hide and seek or if we didn't want to be found by our parents calling us to come home in the evening.

This willow consistently welcomed me in a way no person or thing ever had. I truly felt its joy in my approach. I felt the leaves touch

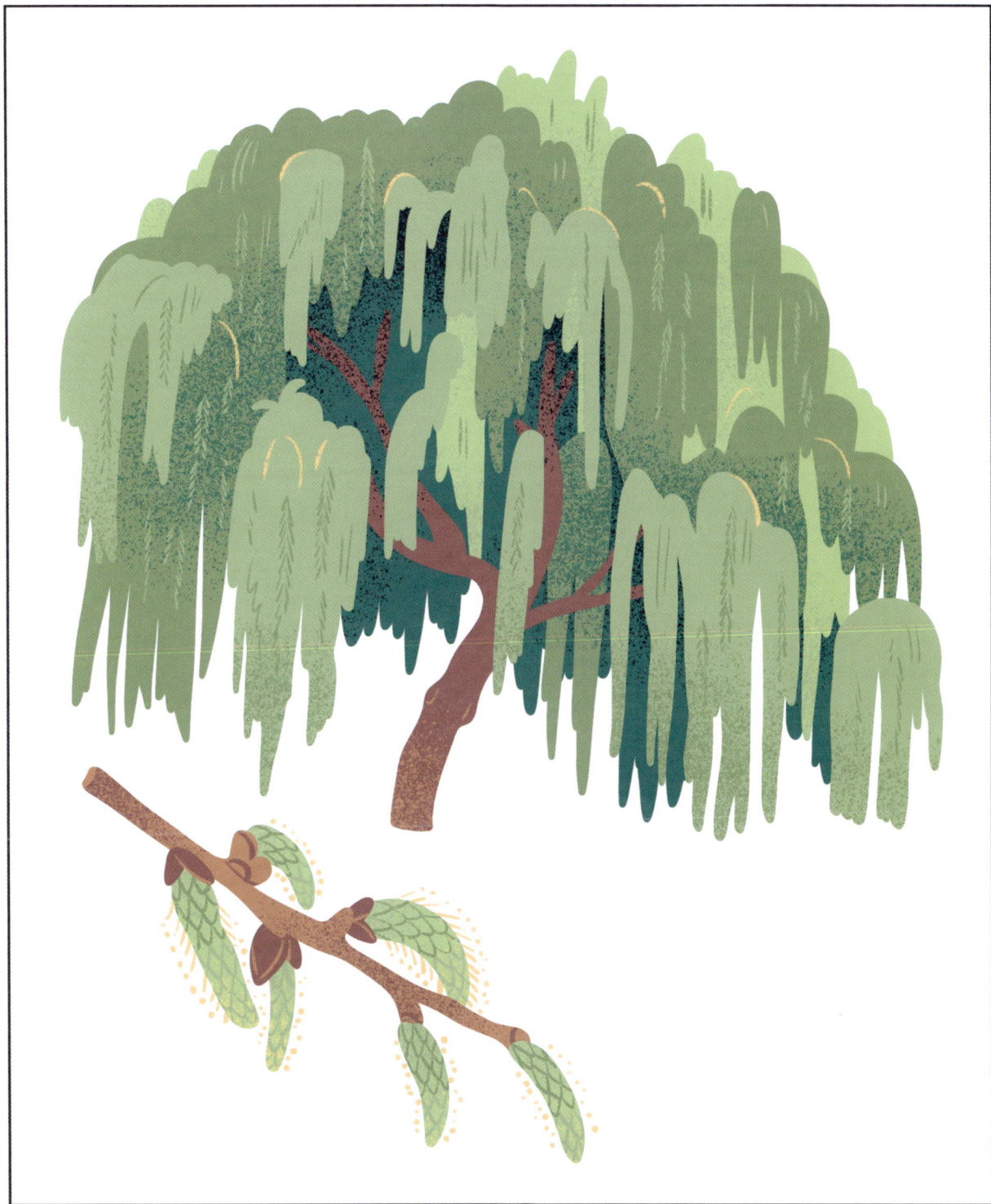

USDA hardiness zones: 4 to 8

Water: water regularly but don't waterlog; once established willows can survive severe flooding

Light requirement: sun to part shade

Soil: moist and well-drained, intolerant to dry soil

Temperature: hardy to -20˚F

Wildlife notes: attracts grazers like rabbits, beavers, deer, and nesting birds

Pollinator friendly: an important larval host plant for butterflies; mining bees detect aromatic compounds emitted by willows, even in minute traces, from far distances

Pests: aphids produce a sugary liquid called "honeydew" that can stain cars parked under infested trees

me as I slowly crossed underneath it, and I'd often wrap myself up in the hanging branches to feel the leaves tickle against my arms, giving me goose bumps. It was like it was willing me to speak, so I began talking to it almost every day. Much like writing in a journal, I verbalized everything I was thinking, going through, struggling with, and excited about. The truth was that after I would visit my willow, I felt better, happier, lighter. When I was young, the equation was simple. When something made me feel good, I wanted more of it. This was perhaps my version of forest bathing. It knew every secret, plan, aspiration of my child and young-adult life, and I continued to visit it well into my adulthood. When my first real medical issue arose at age twenty-six, I sought out the willow for comfort—the place I knew I could retreat to think through my options and emotions. As I got older, I would still sneak into its private sanctuary through the leaves and wrap my arms around it so I could revert to being my six-year-old self. I can still feel the coolness of its bark on my cheek and how my heart softened and relaxed while resting against it. It was here that I came to understand that while we all, us humans, do better when we have a community, some of us can do just as well even if that community isn't human-based.

Before there was aspirin, there was white willow. Salicylates, a group of chemicals found in plants, stop inflammation and reduce pain. Why are they in plants? Probably as a type of defense to help protect from varying diseases and insects. The Sumerians, an ancient civilization of Mesopotamia, recorded the use of salicylates more than 3,000 years ago. In seventeenth century, many of their clay tablets were discovered, some of which had writings

about plant medicine—including the mention of white willow.

Much of our present-day pharmacopeia is derived from the many evolutions of older editions of a pharmacognosy. A pharmacognosy is a book of crude drugs obtained from medicinal plants, animals, fungi, and other natural sources. But it is also the study of searching and making new drugs from natural sources. Aspirin is one such story. Derived from the salicin of white willow, Johann Andreas Buchner, a professor of pharmacology at the University of Munich, isolated, extracted, and purified salicin from the plant. Voilà, the first rendition of aspirin was born. Refining the process took several years. In 1859, professor Hermann Kolbe of Marburg University completed the biochemical structure of salicylic acid and developed the process of making it synthetically. Understanding this history demonstrates how white willow is not the same as aspirin. Aspirin is a synthetic drug made up of acetylsalicylic acid, an isolated and replicated plant constituent that has been concentrated to have a stronger effect. White willow contains salicin, which when ingested converts to salicylic acid and causes an anti-inflammatory effect. But when you take a plant as a whole, you have other constituents working that work like a checks and balances situation. Aspirin is highly potent but can have side effects. White willow might not be as strong as you prefer, but it rarely has side effects and does not lead to stomach bleeding like aspirin can.

So you now have options. You can pop an aspirin, or you can drink a cup of white willow bark tea when you have a headache, back pain, or your arthritis flares up. I usually include it in my cold and flu tea blends to assist with fever and to aid in discomfort. If one of my kids complains of a toothache, we'll simply walk outside to collect a tiny twig from our white willow for them to chew on. It's also great as a gargle for painful sore throats; a strong decoction makes a great wash for bedsores and burns when pain is present.

Here are a few other examples of modern pharmaceuticals derived from plants:

Artemisinin
From *Artemisia annua*, this drug treats multi-drug-resistant malaria

Silymarin
From the seeds of *Silybum marianum*, this drug is used to treat liver disease

Galantamine
An alkaloid extracted from *Galanthus nivalis*, this drug treats Alzheimer's disease

Apomorphine
A semisynthetic morphine derivative, this drug is used in Parkinson's disease

Tiotropium
An atropine derivative from *Atropa belladonna*, this drug is used in chronic obstructive pulmonary disease

White Willow Recipes

INDICATIONS

- Arthritis
- Backache
- Bedsores
- Colds
- Cramping, menstrual
- Diarrhea
- Fever
- Flu
- Gout
- Internal bleeding
- Toothache

*Generally regarded as safe for all populations. Avoid if you have an aspirin allergy; white willow will interact with aspirin, anticoagulants, and antiplatelet medication.

WHITE WILLOW BARK MEDICATED HONEY

Why not add pain-fighting power to your cup of tea? When you blend willow with other natural anti-inflammatories, you've got a power-packed ally to support the aches and pains of whatever the day brings you.

Items needed:
32-oz. glass mason jar
Skewer stick
Fine-mesh strainer

Ingredients:
30 oz. raw, unprocessed honey, ideally from a local beekeeper
3 tbsp. dried white willow bark, cut and sifted
3 tbsp. dried turmeric bark, cut and sifted
1 tbsp. dried ginger root
2 cinnamon sticks

Place all the herbs into the mason jar and pour the honey over the top to fill the jar.

At this point, I often take my skewer stick and poke holes through the herbs to help the honey get all the way to the bottom.

Close up the jar and find a bright, sunny, warm spot for it. Gentle heat helps to extract the medicinal qualities from the herbs.

Every morning and every night, flip your jar over. This means half of the time the jar will be sitting upside down, so ensure your lid is on tight.

Leave for 4 to 6 weeks.

Using your fine-mesh strainer, strain the mixture into any sterilized glass bowl or large measuring cup, then transfer back to your cleaned and sterilized mason jar for storage. Store in a cool and dark place.

Use it on oatmeal as a drizzle or add a teaspoon to tea.

A CORDIAL NIGHTCAP FOR PAIN RELIEF
This nonalcoholic cordial is the perfect sipper before bed to help you ease into pain-free sleep.

Items needed:
8-oz. glass mason jar

Ingredients:
2 tbsp. dried white willow bark
1 tbsp. dried valerian root
½ cinnamon stick
6 to 7 oz. framboise nonalcoholic liqueur

Place all the herbs in the jar, then fill to the top with the framboise.

Close the jar tightly and be sure to label the contents. Give the jar a few good shakes to mix everything up.

Store in a cool, dark place for 3 to 4 weeks, remembering to give it a good shake every day.

Strain and store in a darker colored bottle in a cool, dark place.

Drink ½ to 1 oz. as needed, no more than once a day. Be sure to check in with your healthcare practitioner before use.

Wild Cherry

Prunus avium

Family: Rosaceae
Parts used: bark
Medicinal actions:
anti-inflammatory, anti-spasmodic, antitussive, astringent, circulatory tonic, digestive bitter and tonic, digestive tonic, expectorant, sedative
Native geography:
Europe, Anatolia, Maghreb, and western Asia; now widely distributed across the United States with a high concentration in Oregon and Washington

When I first moved to Portland, Oregon, I lived in a tiny cabin on the back acre of someone's property up in the hills to the west of the city. I say "someone" because I actually never met the owner. The house, a beautifully modernized Craftsman bungalow, sat empty the entire time I lived there. I was attending graduate school at the National University of Natural Medicine. My car had barely made the move down from Bellingham. Now that I think about it, I don't think it ever started again after it reached this destination. I'd probably pep-talked it just enough to get me there. But I had my bike. Biking to NUNM was not the easiest trek, though. These days there is a nice newly paved walkway along Highway 26, but back then you had to merge onto the highway for half a mile before exiting again to reach the southwest city neighborhoods that would eventually dump me down into town. I say "dump me down" because once I reached that southwest neighborhood, it was a joyous ride downhill almost the entire way. And each morning, if it wasn't pissing rain, first I'd look at the sunrise behind Mt. Hood, then I'd reach the cherry blossom trees along the Willamette River before reaching Porter Street. It was an amazing way to start the day. Unfortunately what goes down one way goes up the other; the return trip home was not quite as pleasant.

I've always enjoyed the burn of my lungs on a bike. It feels like I'm clearing out old residue to make room for more breath. And my return ride home definitely kicked in the burn. There were a few breaks of slight downward slopes and plateaus on this trip, but mostly it was up, up, up for four and a half miles. And then just for fun, the steepest, albeit shortest, hill was the road my cabin was on. I joke (but it is true) that my rear end was the best it has ever looked during this time of my life.

I'm not going to sugarcoat the bike commuter lifestyle. There were days when it was raining sideways and I'd show up for class wet and have soggy feet all day. Being a poor grad student, proper rain gear wasn't quite in the budget. Other days, no matter which direction I was going, the wind was against me. The wind! There was always something about it that really got my hackles up. I hated being pushed back by this inevitable force. To be blown upon in such a forceful manner felt personal and rude. I was already working so hard to get to where I was trying to go. The extra resistance was simply unfair.

But I wouldn't have traded those five commuter years for anything. I experience life so much differently from a bike. My state of mind is naturally attuned to its surroundings. I notice the seasons, changes in my neighborhood, and I would interact with people, real live humans, so much more often. It was almost always quicker to get around town on my bike because I wasn't limited in my navigation. I could cut across parks and scoot down a sidewalk or two instead of having to follow one-way roads or getting stuck in traffic. Even after extremely long days and nights, when my mind would trick me into thinking I just couldn't ride, I'd hop on my bike and instantly feel

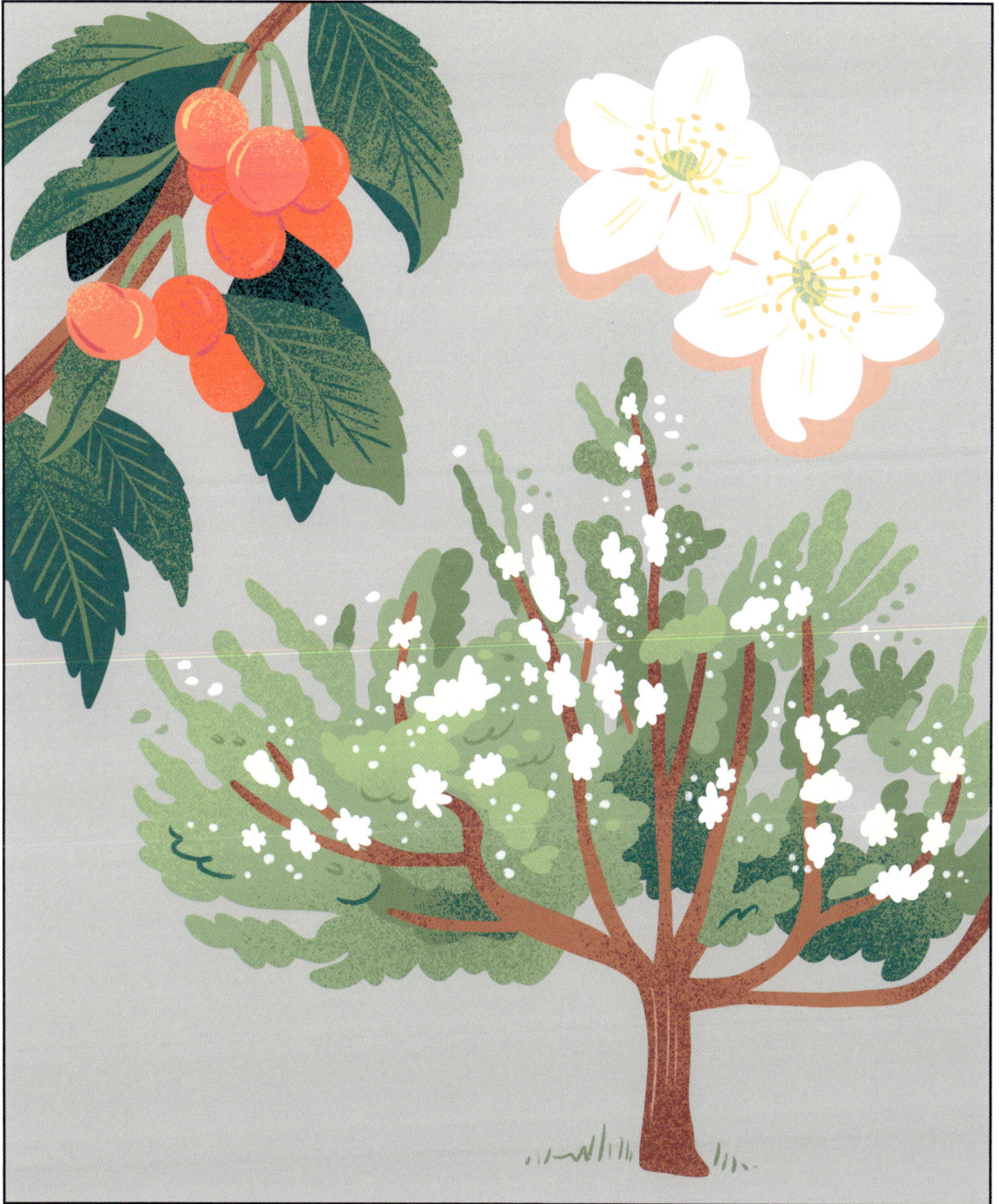

**USDA hardiness
zones:** 3 to 9
Water: water new seedlings every other day
for first two weeks
Light requirement:
full sun
Soil: chalk, clay,
loam, or sand
Temperature: prolonged
spring rains can cause
root damage, while very
dry summers can cause
water stress
Wildlife notes: birds love
wild cherries, especially
thrushes, woodpeckers,
sparrows, bluebirds,
tanagers, orioles, and
cedar waxwings
Pollinator friendly:
attracts bees, beneficial
insects, butterflies,
and moths
Pests: aphids, fruit flies,
sawflies, and scale

revived. My favorite time to ride was on long summer nights, when it felt like I owned the city as I cruised through the quiet streets. While I rode over dark bridges, the water rippled below. On front porches, laughter trickled out from late-night conversations. As I silently glided by, I was witness to so much of what life is, and that always makes me feel happy on the inside.

Another thing that made me happy, giddy even, was springtime bike riding along the Willamette River and experiencing the "snow" of cherry blossoms from the trees that line part of the bank. If you've ever been to Portland, you know the city is divided into east and west by this river. Because of this, there are many bridges that cross the river to connect the city. Twelve of them to be exact, but only nine cross the beautiful downtown waterfront esplanade. This walkway/bikeway runs along either side and is the home of many summer festivals and events that bring the city together. One of the most beloved times on the waterfront isn't a formally structured event, but an event that everyone knows nonetheless. The blooming of the cherry trees that line the esplanade—one hundred of them, perfectly aligned. The trees were a gift from our sister city, Sapporo, Japan, in 1990. This sister city relationship began in 1959 and is one of the longest-standing sister city relationships on record. It continues to be strong, with many citizen and student exchanges, business promotions, festivals, and delegations shared between the two cities.

Living in a city of winter rain can be tough. Everything is wet—all the time. The pros? We don't have to battle snow, our landscapes are never brown, and something is always blooming. But, after slogging in the dampness for many months each year, it is these trees that draw us all together. As they begin to blossom, our hearts are filled with

hope that spring is on the way. As we walk, bike, and take countless photos we embrace these trees as sacred gifts. And if it just so happens to be a bit of a breezy day, it is as if the petals are falling snow, landing in our hair and on our clothes. They seem to be wanting to touch us, just as much as we want to touch them.

—————————

Searching online for info about wild cherry will bring up a lot of controversy about whether it's safe to use or not. In my early herbalist days, there was a lot of misinfor-mation out there that usually took the form of blanket statements that wild cherry was simply not to be used. But as someone who has used wild cherry personally, I knew there had to be more to the story. Like many stone fruits, wild cherry seeds, and to a lesser extent the wilted leaves, hold a concentrated amount of a chemical called amygdalin. Once ingested, this chemical goes through a transformation and ends up as a toxic compound called hydrogen cya-nide. Excess amounts of hydrogen cyanide can wreak havoc very quickly; it basically starves our brain, heart, blood vessels, and lungs of oxygen. But we don't use the seeds in herbal medicine—we use the bark. And in the medicine-making process, the cellular membrane of the bark is disrupted, which drives a conversion toward prussic acid instead of hydrogen cyanide.

However, in large amounts, prussic acid is also toxic. We know this from cattle farmers who have cows that graze on sorghum fields, which can lead to prussic acid poisoning. But Paracelsus's old adage "the poison is in the dose" is where I'm going with wild cherry. Wild cherry bark is an extremely effective cough suppressant. We've all suffered from that very specific, relentless cough at one time or another—it starts as a small tickle, won't stop, and you find yourself needing to leave the room out of embarrassment because your eyes are watering and you can't catch your breath. Or a cough that keeps you up at night when sleep is of vital importance in order to heal. With the correct dosage, prussic acid sedates the cough reflex and opens up the airways. It is also good at drying up excess mucous and creating a productive cough to get lower bronchial phlegm out of the lungs.

While you will most likely only see wild cherry commercially in cold and cough products, it can be a helpful herbal in many other ways. As a naturopathic physician I talk a lot about the digestive system and how to get it to function at its best. One of the most important aspects is getting it to turn "on" before we sit down to eat food. This gives our entire system a head start so that once the food arrives, it is ready to process. Wild cherry bark is classified as a bitter herb, which by definition supports the digestive system. When we have an adequate supply of digestive enzymes, we have a better chance of absorbing nutrients from what we eat and keeping small intestine inflammation low. The sedating nature of prussic acid can also be helpful with acid reflux or GERD, calming the spasms of the lower esophageal sphincter.

In matters of the heart, wild cherry has historically been used to treat cardiac weakness when fluid builds up in the lungs and produces a cough. In this instance, wild cherry acts to nourish and tone the heart muscle as well as to reestablish balance in the circulatory system.

Currently *Prunus avium* is listed on the invasive species list. Birds and other animals carry and drop the seeds, which are quick to self-seed, so I suggest wildcrafting rather than cultivating this plant. Search for a downed tree or branches after a windstorm rather than peeling bark directly off a living tree if it can be avoided. I suggest using a peeling spud (sometimes called a debarking spud), which is a tool that removes the bulk of the bark by prying it off. Once it is removed, you can use a peeler to scrape off the inner bark, which is the medicinal part.

Wild Cherry Recipes

INDICATIONS

- Asthma
- Bloating
- Bronchitis
- Colds
- Coughs
- Digestion tonic
- GERD
- Heart palpitations
- Heart weakness with cough
- High blood pressure

If dosed correctly, generally regarded as safe for all populations. Avoid if pregnant.

WILD CHERRY BARK COUGH SYRUP

I never go through winter without having this syrup on hand. A cough is one of those symptoms you need to nip in the bud, as it's opportunistic. If left untreated, a cough can make its way insidiously to the lower recess of the lungs, where it loves to wreak havoc. Thankfully this syrup tastes good and packs a powerful punch.

Items needed:
Stockpot
Mason jar
Stirring spoon
Fine-mesh strainer
Storage bottles

Ingredients:
4 tbsp. dried wild cherry bark
2 tbsp. dried elecampane root
2 tbsp. dried marshmallow root
1 tbsp. dried rosemary leaf
1 tbsp. dried mullein leaf
64 oz. water + 8 oz. for marshmallow extraction
3 cups organic cane sugar
½ cup apple cider vinegar

Put the water, wild cherry bark, and elecampane root into the stockpot and bring up to a simmer. Simmer on low with the lid off for 10 minutes, then bring to a low boil. Boil until the water is reduced by half. Turn off the heat and add the rosemary and mullein. Cover and let it all steep for 1 hour.

In the meantime, put the marshmallow into the mason jar and pour 8 oz. of room-temperature water over it. Let steep for 1 hour.

Strain the marshmallow and the stockpot mixtures, then transfer everything back to the stockpot.

Bring it back up to a low boil and boil for 10 minutes, reducing it slightly.

Once you have approximately 28 oz. of liquid left, add the sugar and boil until dissolved, stirring often. Turn off the heat and let it cool for 20 minutes. Add in the apple cider vinegar and give it a stir.

Cool completely, then transfer to storage bottles and keep in the refrigerator.

WILD CHERRY BARK FUDGE

I will put herbs in anything and I am a self-proclaimed chocoholic, so this recipe satisfies both my desires. When you are on the illness-recovery train, sometimes a touch of sweetness really hits the spot, too.

Items needed:
Mixing bowl
8-x-8-inch baking pan

Ingredients:
1 cup cacao powder
4 tbsp. smooth nut or seed butter of your choice
2 tbsp. coconut oil, melted
2 tbsp. wild cherry bark, ground
6 tbsp. raw honey
2 tsp. lemon zest
2 pinches sea salt

First, mix together the cacao, nut butter, oil, wild cherry bark, honey, lemon, and salt. Mix until everything is combined and has a thick but still workable consistency. If it is too thick, add a bit more honey.

Line the bottom of the baking pan with parchment paper. Transfer the chocolate to the pan and put another piece of parchment on top. Using a small rolling pin (or anything you can think of to flatten out the chocolate in the pan), smooth it to roughly ¼ inch in thickness.

Pull off the top piece of parchment and sprinkle the dough with sea salt, cacao, or more lemon zest.

Be sure to cut the pan's contents into bars at this point—before you freeze it.

Put into the freezer and chill for 1 hour. Store in the refrigerator and eat within 2 weeks, or store in the freezer and pull out bars one at a time to share.

Appendices

Herbal Terms

Science loves chemistry and classification. In a laboratory, one of the ways scientists study plant medicine is to isolate the different chemical components within a plant. In doing so they are identifying all of the chemical "actions" each plant possesses. A few examples would be a tannin, which is a polyphenolic biomolecule with a carbohydrate backbone and a phenol, an organic compound consisting of a benzene ring with a hydroxyl group. Tannins are known to produce an astringent action and phenols inhibit enzymes that often lead to disease. Knowing these terms gives you the language of a scientist and promotes a deeper learning of plant chemistry. If you love this part of science, you'll enjoy reading the listed most common plant constituents below.

But if all of this talk of chemistry tends to make your head swim, not to worry. Herbalism uses simple terms to describe how plants affect the physical body. For the purposes of this book I've stuck to these terms when describing each tree's medicinal action potential. If you study and learn these terms they can become a tool when talking about herbal medicine and help you to better describe your thoughts and feelings about them.

Adaptogens are strengthening herbs that help us adapt to stress by interacting with the endocrine system.

Alteratives are herbs that that produce a gradual beneficial change in the body by improving nutrition and eliminating metabolic waste via the liver.

Analgesics are medications that are applied internally or externally to reduce pain.

Anthelmintic plants kill or assist in the expulsion of intestinal worms.

Anti-inflammatory herbs reduce inflammation in the body.

Antimicrobials are herbs that interfere with the proliferation and life cycle of microbes: bacteria, fungi, and viruses.

Anodynes are herbs that relieve pain.

Antioxidant substances protect against oxidation and degradation from free radical damage.

Antirheumatic medicines prevent or relieve rheumatic symptoms such as joint pains, limited mobility, and swelling.

Antispasmodic plants reduce or relieve smooth muscle spasms.

Antitussives are substances that reduces the amount of or severity of coughing.

Aphrodisiac herbs are those that nourish, build, and stimulate sexual desire and potency.

Astringents draw tissues together, tightening and toning them to reduce secretions and discharge.

Bitters stimulate digestion by enhancing digestive secretion and peristaltic movements of the gut.

Bronchodilator plants cause widening of the bronchi.

Cardiacs are herbs that stimulate or otherwise positively affect the heart.

Carminative herbs are high in essential oils and help ease digestion by relieving gas, spasms, and cramps.

Cholagogues and **choleretics** promote the production of bile in the liver.

Demulcents are soothing mucilaginous herbs that can be taken internally to soothe and protect damaged or inflamed tissue.

Depurative substances improve detoxification and aid elimination to reduce the accumulation of metabolic waste products.

Diaphoretics are herbs that cause sweating by increasing circulation in the periphery of the body.

Diuretics are herbs that stimulate the flow of urine and help remove fluids from the body.

Emetics are herbs that promote vomiting.

Emmenagogues are herbs that stimulate and promote menstruation.

Expectorants are herbs that assist the body in expelling mucous from the upper respiratory tract.

Febrifuge or antipyretic plants reduce or prevent fever.

Galactagogues are herbs that encourage the flow of breast milk.

Hemostatics are herbs that stop bleeding.

Hepatics are herbs that generally support liver function.

Hypnotics and sedatives are plants that promote relaxation and deep sleep.

Hypolipidemics are herbs that mildly reduce serum lipids, including triglycerides and cholesterol.

Hypotensives act to reduce high blood pressure.

Immunomodulators restore balance to a dysfunctional immune system.

Immunostimulants stimulate the immune system to protect against infection.

Laxative herbs are those that stimulate or promote bowel movements in a gentle way.

Mucilaginous herbs are ones that produce a gelatinous consistency.

Nervines are herbs that soothe the nervous system. They can stimulate, nourish, or sedate.

Purgatives are herbs that promote bowel expulsion in a rapid and quick manner.

Relaxant plants promote relaxation and can reduce tension.

Rubefacients are applied externally and cause a mild local irritation and draw blood to the area through capillary dilation.

Sedatives are often a subcategory of nervines that decrease nervous tension.

Sialogogues are herbs that stimulate the production of saliva.

Stimulant substances raise levels of physiological or nervous activity in the body.

Stomachics promote the appetite or assist digestion.

Tonics are herbs that bring tone to an organ or tissue and/or generally improve function to a particular system.

Uterine tonics are substances that increase the tone of the uterine muscle.

Vasoconstrictors narrow the blood vessels, which can raise blood pressure.

Vasodilators are substances that dilate the blood vessels.

Vulneraries are wound-healing herbs used internally and externally.

Plant Chemistry Terms

Alkaloids have one nitrogen atom within a cyclic structure, typically in an amine-like form, reduce palatability, healing agents.

Bitters have a wide variety of chemical structures, and stimulate a reflex action through the tastebuds that stimulates digestive function.

Coumarin is a benzene molecule with two adjacent hydrogen atoms replaced by an unsaturated lactone ring; it is an anticoagulant.

Flavonoids have a 15-carbon skeleton with two benzene rings which each have 6 carbons and the connecting bridge has 3 carbons; they have a wide range of functions.

Lignins have a non-crystalline (amorphous) structure due to its highly complex branched configuration. They reduce digestibility. Late maturity forage has more lignin, is less palatable.

Saponins are composed of a complex glycoside with a polycyclic carbon skeleton linked to one or more sugar units. They are strongly anti-inflammatory, but can cause bloat.

Tannins have multiple phenol groups attached to a carbohydrate backbone, typically a glucose molecule. A strong astringent, they reduce palatability.

Volatile oils are a complex mixture of organic compounds primarily composed of terpenes. Are antiseptic, stimulating, and act on the central nervous system.

Sources and Further Reading

SOURCES

Introduction
Engermann, K., Bocker, P., and Arge, L. "Residential Green Space in Childhood Is Associated with Lower Risk of Psychiatric Disorders from Adolescence into Adulthood." *PNAS*, 116 (11) (February 25, 2019): 5188-93. https://doi.org/10.1073/pnas.1807504116.

Acacia
Sadiq M.B., Tarning J., Aye Cho T.Z., and Anal A.K. "Antibacterial Activities and Possible Modes of Action of *Acacia nilotica* (L.) Del. against Multidrug-Resistant *Escherichia coli* and Salmonella." *Molecules* 22(1). (January 14, 2017): 47. doi: 10.3390/molecules22010047. PMID: 28098806; PMCID: PMC6155900.

Banyan
Chandrasekar, S.B., Bhanumathy, M., Pawar, A. T., Somasundaram, T., "Phytopharmacology of *Ficus religiosa*," *Pharmacognosy Reviews* 4(8) (2010): 195-9. https://doi:10.4103/0973-7847.70918, PMCID: PMC3249921PMID: 22228961.

Beech
Connell, W. F., Johnston, Grant M., and Boyd, Eldon M. "On the Expectorant Action of Resyl and Other Guaiacols." *Canadian Medical Association Journal*. March 1940; 42(3): 220-23. http://www.ncbi.nlm.nih.gov/pmc/articles/PMC537807/.

Parker, A. C. "Iroquois Uses of Maize and Other Food Plants." *Education Department Bulletin*, University of the State of New York, 482 (1910). Albany, New York. https://archive.org/details/iroquoisusesofma00parkrich.

California Bay Laurel
Carranza, M.G., Sevigny, M.B., Banerjee, D., Fox-Cubley, L. "Antibacterial activity of native California medicinal plant extracts isolated from *Rhamnus californica* and *Umbellularia californica*." *Annals of Clinical Microbiology and Antimicrobials*, 14 (29) (May 23, 2015).

https://doi:10.1186/s12941-015-0086-0. PMID: 26001558; PMCID: PMC4443625.

Crab Apple
Xiangquan Zeng, He Li,Weibo Jiang, Qianqian Li, Yu Xi, Xiaomei Wang, Jian Li. "Phytochemical compositions, health-promoting properties and food applications of crabapples: A review." *Food Chemistry* (2022). https://doi:10.1016/j.foodchem.2022.132789.

Eucalyptus
Anonymous. "The Trees That Captured California." *Sunset* August 1956: 44-49.

Margolin, Louis. "Eucalyptus Culture in Hawaii." Hawaii Board of Agriculture and Forestry, Division of Forestry, in cooperation with USDA Forest Service. 1911: 80. Honolulu, HI.

Ginkgo
Gachowska M, Szlasa W, Saczko J, Kulbacka J. Neuroregulatory role of ginkgolides. *Molecular Biology Reports* 48(7) (2021):5689-97. doi: 10.1007/s11033-021-06535-2. PMID: 34245409; PMCID: PMC8338821.

Silberstein, R.B., Pipingas, A., Song, J., Camfield, D.A., Nathan, P.J., Stough, C. "Examining brain-cognition effects of ginkgo biloba extract: brain activation in the left temporal and left prefrontal cortex in an object working memory task." *Evidence-Based Complementary and Alternative Medicine* (2011): 164139. https://doi:10.1155/2011/164139. PMID: 21941584; PMCID: PMC3166615.

Zhang, H.F., Huang, L.B., Zhong, Y.B., Zhou, Q.H., Wang, H.L., Zheng, G.Q., Lin, Y. An. "Overview of Systematic Reviews of Ginkgo biloba Extracts for Mild Cognitive Impairment and Dementia." *Frontiers in Aging Neuroscience* 8. (2016):276. https://doi:10.3389/fnagi.2016.00276. PMID: 27999539; PMCID: PMC5138224.

Hawthorn
Tassell, M.C, Kingston, R., Gilroy, D., Lehane, M., Furey, A. "Hawthorn (*Crataegus* spp.) in the treatment of

cardiovascular disease." *Pharmacogn Rev.*, 4 (7). (January 2010): 32–41. https://doi:10.4103/0973-7847.65324. PMID: 22228939; PMCID: PMC3249900.

Cloud, A., Vilcins, D., McEwen, B. "The effect of hawthorn (*Crataegus* spp.) on blood pressure: A systematic review." *Advances in Integrative Medicine* 7, Issue 3 (2020): 167–75. ISSN 2212-9588. https://doi.org/10.1016/j.aimed.2019.09.002.

Juniper
Little Jr., Elbert L. *Checklist of United States Trees (Native and Naturalized): Agricultural Handbook 541.* U.S. Department of Agriculture, Forest Service. 1979.

Mozingo, Hugh N. *Shrubs of the Great Basin: A Natural History.* University of Nevada Press. 1987.

Larch
Hauer, J., and Anderer, F.A. "Mechanism of stimulation of human natural killer cytotoxicity by arabinogalactan from *Larix occidentalis*." *Cancer Immunology, Immunotherapy* 36 (4) (1993): 237–44. https://doi: 10.1007/BF01740905. PMID: 8439987; PMCID: PMC11038192.

Kelly, G. "Ara 6: Larch Arabinogalactan." (2023) https://www.dadamo.com/txt/index.pl?1028

Riede, L., Grube, B., Gruenwald, J. "Larch arabinogalactan effects on reducing incidence of upper respiratory infections." *Current Medical Research and Opinion* 29 no. 3 (2013): 251–58. https://doi: 10.1185/03007995.2013.765837. PMID: 23339578.

Shin-ichi Koizumi, Kazutaka Masuko, Daiko Wakita, et.al, "Extracts of *Larix leptolepis* effectively augments the generation of tumor antigen-specific cytotoxic T lymphocytes via activation of dendritic cells in TLR-2 and TLR-4-dependent manner." *Cellular Immunology* 276 (1-2) (2012): 153–61. ISSN 0008-8749. https://doi.org/10.1016/j.cellimm.2012.05.002.

London Plane Tree
Hajhashemi ,V., Ghannadi, A., Mousavi, S. "Antinociceptive study of extracts of *Platanus orientalis* leaves in mice." *Res. Pharm. Sci.* 6 (2). (2011):123–8. PMID: 22224096; PMCID: PMC324.9775.

Yesilada, E, Akkol, E.K., Aydin, A., Hamitoğlu, M. "A Realistic Approach for Anti-Inflammatory, Antinociceptive and Antimutagenic Activities, and Risk Assessment of the Aqueous Extract of *Platanus orientalis* L. Leaves." *Current Molecular Pharmacology.* 14 (5) (2021):753–59. https://doi: 10.2174/1874467214999210011220358. PMID: 33430755.

Magnolia
Faysal, Md., Khan, J., Zehravi, M, et. al, 2023/11/24, "Neuropharmacological potential of honokiol and its derivatives from Chinese herb *Magnolia* species: understandings from therapeutic viewpoint" *Chinese Medicine* 18 (154) (2023). https://doi.org/10.1186/s13020-023-00846-1.

Poivre, M., Duez, P. "Biological activity and toxicity of the Chinese herb *Magnolia officinalis* Rehder & E. Wilson (Houpo) and its constituents." Journal of Zhejiang University 18 (3) (2017):194–214. https://doi: 10.1631/jzus.B1600299. PMID: 28271656; PMCID: PMC5365644.

Tsai, S.K., Huang, S.S., Hong, C.Y. "Myocardial protective effect of honokiol: an active component in Magnolia officinalis." *Planta Medica* 62 (6) (1996):503–6. https://doi: 10.1055/s-2006-957957. PMID: 9000881.

Maple
Fan, Y., Lin, F., Zhang, R., Wang, M., Gu, R., Long, C. "*Acer truncatum* Bunge: A comprehensive review on ethnobotany, phytochemistry and pharmacology." *Journal of Ethnopharmacolology.* 282 (2022):114572. https://doi: 10.1016/j.jep.2021.114572. PMID: 34487848.

Liya Li, Hang Ma, Tingting Liu, Zhanjun Ding, Wei Liu, Qiong Gu, Yu Mu, Jun Xu, Navindra P. Seeram, Xueshi Huang, Jialin Xu. "Glucitol-core containing gallotannins-enriched red maple (*Acer rubrum*) leaves extract alleviated obesity via modulating short-chain fatty acid production in high-fat diet-fed mice." *Journal of Functional Foods* 70 (2020). ISSN 1756-4646, https://doi.org/10.1016/j.jff.2020.103970.

Tae woo Oh, Hyun Ju Do, Kwang-Youn Kim, Kwang Il Park, Jin Yeul Ma. "Leaves of *Acer palmatum thumb.* Rescues N-ethyl-N-nitrosourea (ENU)-Induced retinal degeneration in mice." *Phytomedicine* 42 (2018): 51–55, ISSN 0944-7113, https://doi.org/10.1016/j.phymed.2018.03.026.

Zhu LB, Zhang YC, Huang HH, Lin J. "Prospects for clinical applications of butyrate-producing bacteria." *World Journal of Clinical Pediatrics.* 10 (5) (2021):84–92. https://doi:10.5409/wjcp.v10.i5.84. PMID: 34616650; PMCID: PMC8465514.

Noni
Palu, A., Deng, S., West, B., Jensen, J. "Xanthine oxidase inhibiting effects of noni (*Morinda citrifolia*) fruit juice." *Phytotherapy Research.* 23 (12) (2009):1790–1. https://doi:10.1002/ptr.2842. PMID: 19434757.

Pine
Chiavaroli, A., Di Simone, S.C., Acquaviva, A., Libero, M.L., Campana, C., Recinella, L., Leone, S., Brunetti, L., Orlando, G., Nilofar, V.I., Cesa, S., Zengin, G., Menghini, L., Ferrante, C. "Protective Effects of PollenAid Plus Soft Gel Capsules' Hydroalcoholic Extract in Isolated Prostates and Ovaries Exposed to Lipopolysaccharide." *Molecules* 27 (19) (2022): 6279. https://doi: 10.3390/molecules27196279. PMID: 36234818; PMCID: PMC9570715.

Giachi, G., Pallecchi, P., Romualdi, A., Ribechini, E., Lucejko, J.J., Colombini, M.P., Mariotti Lippi, M. "Ingredients of a 2,000-y-old medicine revealed by chemical, mineralogical, and botanical investigations." *Proceedings of the National Academy of Sciences of the USA.* 110 (4) (203):1193–6. https://doi:10.1073/pnas.1216776110. PMID: 23297212; PMCID: PMC3557061.

Liang, S.B., Liang, N., Bu, F.L., Lai, B.Y., Zhang, Y.P., Cao, H.J., Fei, Y.T., Robinson, N., Liu, J.P. "The Potential Effects and Use of Chinese Herbal Medicine Pine Pollen (*Pinus pollen*): A Bibliometric Analysis of Pharmacological and Clinical Studies." *World Journal of Traditional Chinese Medicine* 6 (2) (2020):163–70. https://doi: 10.4103/wjtcm.wjtcm_4_20. PMID: 34327226; PMCID: PMC8318335.

Liu, X. "Anti-fatigue function of pine pollen." *Chinese Journal of Biochemical Pharmaceutics* (2004). CDC, Jiangsu Province, China. Original translation by RAW Forest Foods.

Luo, Y., Wei, Y., Wang, T., Chen, D., Lu, T., Wu, R., Si, K. "Pine pollen inhibits cell apoptosis-related protein expression in the cerebral cortex of mice with arsenic poisoning." *Neural Regeneration Research* 7 (12) (2012):896–9. https://doi:10.3969/j.issn.1673-5374.2012.12.003. PMID: 25722672; PMCID: PMC4341283.

Shang, H., Niu, X., Cui, W., et al. "Anti-tumor activity of polysaccharides extracted from *Pinus massoniana* pollen in colorectal cancer: in vitro and in vivo studies." *Food and Function* 13 (11) (2022):6350–61. https://doi:10.1039/d1fo03908c.

Poplar
Kis, B., Avram, S., Pavel, I. Z., Lombrea, A., Buda, V., Dehelean, C. A., Soica, C., Yerer, M. B., Bojin, F., Folescu, R., & Danciu, C. (2020). "Recent Advances Regarding the Phytochemical and Therapeutic Uses of *Populus nigra* L. Buds." *Plants* 9 (11). (2020): 1,464. https://doi.org/10.3390/plants9111464.

Patel, S.K., Surowiec, S.M. "Intermittent Claudication." *StatPearls* (2023). https://www.ncbi.nlm.nih.gov/books/NBK430778/.

Savage, K., Firth, J., Stough, C., Sarris, J. "GABA-modulating phytomedicines for anxiety: A systematic review of preclinical and clinical evidence." *Phytotherapy Research.* 32 (1) (2018):3–18. https://doi:10.1002/ptr.5940. PMID: 29168225.

Sitka Spruce
Jyske, T., Järvenpää, E., Kunnas, S., Sarjala, T., Raitanen, J.E., Mäki, M., Pastell, H., Korpinen, R., Kaseva, J., Tupasela, T. "Sprouts and Needles of Norway Spruce (*Picea abies* (L.) Karst.) as Nordic Specialty-Consumer Acceptance, Stability of Nutrients, and Bioactivities during Storage." *Molecules* 25 (18) (2020):4,187. https://doi:10.3390/molecules25184187. PMID: 32932686; PMCID: PMC7570650.

White Willow
Grandstaff, G., Kuzovkina, Y.A., Legrand, A. "Attraction of Bees to Native and Introduced Willows (Salix spp.)." *Forests* 14 (5) (2023):959. https://doi.org/10.3390/f14050959.

Wild Cherry
Grandjean, P. "Paracelsus Revisited: The Dose Concept in a Complex World." *Basic Clinical Pharmacology & Toxicology* 119 (2) (2016):126-32. https://doi:10.1111/bcpt.12622. PMID: 27214290; PMCID: PMC4942381.

Teixeira, Essenfelder L., Gomes, A.A., Coimbra, J.L.M., Moreira, M.A., Ferraz, S.M., Miquelluti D.J., Felippe da Silva, G., Magalhães, M.L.B. "Salivary β-glucosidase as a direct factor influencing the occurrence of halitosis." *Biochemistry and Biophysics Reports* 26 (2021):100965. https://doi:10.1016/j.bbrep.2021.100965. PMID: 33732903; PMCID: PMC7941027.

Telichowska, A., Kobus-Cisowska, J., Szulc, P. "Phytopharmacological Possibilities of Bird Cherry *Prunus padus* L. and *Prunus serotina* L. Species and Their Bioactive Phytochemicals." *Nutrients* 12 (7) (2020):1,966. https://doi:10.3390/nu12071966. PMID: 32630652; PMCID: PMC7399899.

FURTHER READING

Arvigo, R., and Epstein, N. *Rainforest Home Remedies.* HarperCollins, 2001.

Beresford-Kroeger, D. *To Speak for the Trees: My Life's Journey from Ancient Celtic Wisdom to a Healing Vision of the Forest.* Timber Press, 2021.

Bone, K. *A Clinical Guide to Blending Liquid Herbs: Herbal Formulations for the Individual Patient.* Elsevier Science, 2003.

Conway, P. *Tree Medicine: A Comprehensive Guide to the Healing Power of Over 150 Trees.* Judy Piatkus Publishing, 2002.

Kloos, S. *Pacific Northwest Medicinal Plants: Identify, Harvest, and Use 120 Wild Herbs for Health and Wellness.* Timber Press, 2017.

Lust, J. *The Herb Book: The Most Complete Catalog of Herbs Ever Published.* Dover, 2014.

Phillips, N. and M., *The Herbalist's Way: The Art and Practice of Healing with Plant Medicines.* Chelsea Green Publishing, 2005.

Romm, A. *Botanical Medicine for Women's Health.* Elsevier, 2018.

Torbyn, G., Denham, A., and Whitelegg, M. *The Western Herbal Tradition: 2000 Years of Traditional Plant Knowledge.* Churchill Livingstone, 2011.

Acknowledgments

Many years ago, I found myself lost in the 5,200 acres of Forest Park, just northwest of downtown Portland, Oregon. I had traversed the trails of this park for years but on this particular day, I must have been distracted by my thoughts. It was the holiday season, and I was pet-sitting two dogs for friends. What started out as a boisterous adventure suddenly turned concerning as I realized I was disoriented. I knew the sun would sets at about 4:30p.m. in December, which meant I had approximately 45 minutes to get back to my car. The dogs had already sensed that something was off; instead of running free to explore the bushes and trees, they began acting protective, positioning themselves one in front of me and the other behind. At one point, I even slid down part of an unrecognized hill in an attempt to connect with the trail. The dogs looked skeptical but eventually followed. I didn't wind up where I had hoped, but I did find myself standing among a mesmerizing grove of trees. Had I been here before? As I stood there, wondering what to do, a chorus of voices rose up around me. The trees were offering me a gift. A gift of connection, of stories centuries old, and secrets of the forest. I felt frozen in time, yet at the same time felt a lifetime of wisdom wash over me. They swayed, sang, and praised as I watched in reverence. What a gift to be offered. I hardly felt worthy. "But what can I offer in return," I asked. The answer was swift and clear: *Be our voice so that others can heal.*

Trees have interjected themselves in my life so often, I would be foolish to not believe in their guiding power. As a child, they were my refuge. As a struggling youth, I would escape by hiding in them. Random strangers have led me to must-see mystical orchards, and new friends have shared their lore around campfires. More times than not, I've taken detours on road trips for the sake of seeing a tree, a forest, or some thicket that someone had mentioned in passing. I've always answered the call. Because, why not?

A special thanks to my editor, Stacee Lawrence, who, like me, acknowledges a fascination with the natural world and our place in it. Thank you for always trusting me, and seeing something in me that can be hard for me to see in myself. Brian Benson, wow do I feel lucky to have followed my intuition, which led me to you! You're a gifted writer and teacher, and it was such an honor to have you edit my stories. And to all of my peers who shared the cozy "attic" each and every Thursday: Alec, Ali, Cate, Kati, Katie aka Oscar, Sage and Sara. Thank you, thank you, thank you. To share and exchange our work in such a safe environment was the highlight of my fall 2023 season. Saso, a special thank-you to you. You were the first person to instill in me that my stories are worth sharing. You pushed to hear more, and it allowed me to recognize that I do have something of worth to share.

And last but not least, thanks to my family. Thank you for indulging me with my witchy, wild-woman ways. May our lives be deeply rooted but our branches be ever intertwined, and always reaching to the stars. .

ABOUT THE AUTHOR

Combining science, herbs, and natural medicine, Dr. JJ Pursell has dedicated her life to helping others be the healthiest they can be. She earned her doctorate in naturopathy and her master's in acupuncture in 2007 from the National University of Natural Medicine in Portland, Oregon. But her love of botanical medicine has always been a part of her life. Influenced by her dad's flower farm and her years as an herbal apprentice, working with herbal medicines has been more of a calling than a profession.

She is currently pursuing her PhD in the cross-cultural examination of mystical states for initiation, healing, and tribal decision-making. She also has a private medical practice and legally facilitates psilocybin sessions in Oregon. When she isn't making medicine, teaching, or writing, you'll find her putzing around her garden, checking in on her bees, and enjoying every minute she can with her family.